Duchenne Muscular Dystrophy

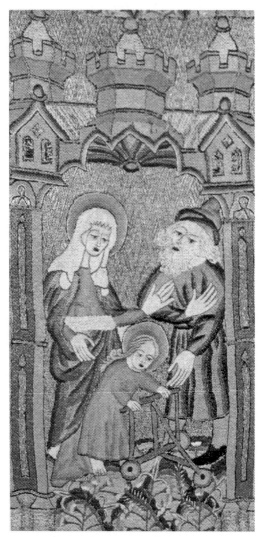

Detail of an orphery on a fourteenth century dalmatic in The Burrell Collection, Glasgow. See colour plate section in the centre of this book.

Duchenne Muscular Dystrophy

THIRD EDITION

By

Alan E.H. Emery
Emeritus Professor of Human Genetics
  University of Edinburgh
  UK
Honorary Visiting Fellow
  Green College, Oxford
  UK

Francesco Muntoni
Professor in Pediatric Neurology
  Director, Dubowitz Neuromuscular Centre
  Department of Paediatrics
  Imperial College London
  UK

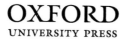

OXFORD
UNIVERSITY PRESS

*This book has been printed digitally and produced in a standard specification
in order to ensure its continuing availability*

OXFORD
UNIVERSITY PRESS

Great Clarendon Street, Oxford OX2 6DP

Oxford University Press is a department of the University of Oxford.
It furthers the University's objective of excellence in research, scholarship,
and education by publishing worldwide in

Oxford New York

Auckland Cape Town Dar es Salaam Hong Kong Karachi
Kuala Lumpur Madrid Melbourne Mexico City Nairobi
New Delhi Shanghai Taipei Toronto
With offices in
Argentina Austria Brazil Chile Czech Republic France Greece
Guatemala Hungary Italy Japan South Korea Poland Portugal
Singapore Switzerland Thailand Turkey Ukraine Vietnam

Oxford is a registered trade mark of Oxford University Press
in the UK and in certain other countries

Published in the United States
by Oxford University Press Inc., New York

© Oxford University Press, 2003

ISBN 0-19-851531-6

Printed and bound by CPI Antony Rowe, Eastbourne

Preface

The first edition of this book was being written in the mid-1980s, at a time when the gene for Duchenne muscular dystrophy was first localized and later isolated and characterized. The defective protein in the disease, later named *dystrophin*, proved to be located in the muscle membrane. This finding resulted in subsequent ideas of pathogenesis moving away from previous notions of a possible neurogenic or vascular origin of the disease to a structural defect in the muscle membrane. Furthermore, the technology used in the disease to characterize the defective gene and its product, now referred to as positional cloning, was subsequently applied to many other genetic disorders including other forms of muscular dystrophy. In fact the molecular bases of some 30 different forms of dystrophy are now recognized, though not all the protein defects have proved to be localized to the sarcolemma. These findings now provide the laboratory basis for establishing a precise diagnosis in an affected individual as well as for reliable genetic counselling and prenatal diagnosis. But many problems still remain, not least the need for a clearer understanding of the details of pathogenesis which is essential if a logical approach to an effective drug treatment is ever to be found. The care of affected children is also changing. A more positive approach is clearly developing, including new approaches to the management of respiratory and cardiac problems and new possibilities in gene therapy.

It is a great pleasure for us to thank our many colleagues for providing suggestions and much useful information. In this regard we are particularly grateful to Dr Adnan Manzur, Paediatrician and Paediatric Neurologist at the Hammersmith Hospital, London, for his help in the chapter on treatment and management. We also wish to thank Professor Caroline Sewry and Dr Sue Brown, Dubowitz Neuromuscular Unit at the Hammersmith Hospital, for their help with the pathology illustrations and the Chapter on pathogenesis, respectively.

Finally, we have endeavoured to bring the information as up-to-date as possible, though without ignoring earlier important findings. It is our sincere hope that all those involved with the diagnosis, care, and treatment of this disorder from the laboratory to the bedside and community will find the book useful.

Oxford/Exeter   A.E.H.E.
London   F.M.
2003

Contents

Abbreviations

AAV	adeno-associated virus
ACE	angiotensin-converting enzyme
ADP	adenosine diphosphate
AMP	adenosine monophosphate
ATP	adenosine triphosphate
bFGF	basic fibroblast growth factor
BMD	Becker type muscular dystrophy
CK	creatine kinase
cM	centimorgan
CT	computerized tomography
DAPC	dystrophin-associated glycoprotein complex
DEXA	dual-energy X-ray absorptiometry
DMD	Duchenne muscular dystrophy
DOVAMS	detection of virtually all mutations system
ECG	electrocardiogram
EEG	electroencephalography
EMG	electromyography
ENMC	European Neuromuscular Centre
FIGE	field inversion gel electrophoresis
FKRP	Fukutin-related protein
FVC	forced vital capacity
GABA	γ-aminobutyric acid
GLUT4	glucose transporter 4
GOT	glutamic-oxaloacetic transaminase
GPT	glutamic-pyruvic transaminase
Grb2	growth factor receptor bound 2 (protein)
HFDR	high-frequency deletion region
HFMD	hypertrophic feline muscular dystrophy

HLA	human leukocyte antigen (system)
IGF	insulin-like growth factor
IL1RAPL1	interleukin-1 receptor related protein
IU	international units
KAFO	knee ankle foot orthoses
kb	kilobase
LDH	lactate dehydrogenase
LGMD	limb girdle muscular dystrophy
MAPK	mitogen-activated protein kinase
MDC1A	muscular dystrophy congenital 1A (also MDC1B, MDC1C, etc.)
MRI	magnetic resonance imaging
MRS	magnetic resonance spectroscopy
MW	molecular weight
MZ	monozygotic
NADP	nicotinamide–adenine dinucleotide phosphate
NIPPV	nasal intermittent positive pressure ventilation
NMR	nuclear magnetic resonance
nNOS	neuronal nitric oxide synthase
NOS	nitric oxide synthase
ORF	open reading frame
OTC	ornithine transcarbamylase
PABP2	poly A binding protein 2
pCO_2	arterial carbon dioxide tension
PCR	polymerase chain reaction
PERT	phenol-enhanced reassociation technique
PFGE	pulsed-field gel electrophoresis
PK	pyruvate kinase
pO_2	arterial oxygen tension
PTT	protein truncation test

RFLPs	restriction fragment length polymorphisms	SMA	spinal muscular atrophy
RNA	ribonucleic acid	SNPs	single nucleotide polymorphisms
SAPK3	stress-activated protein kinase-3	SSCP	single-strand conformation polymorphism
SCARMD	severe childhood onset autosomal recessive muscular dystrophy	TGF-β	transforming growth factor β
SCK	serum creatine kinase	XLDCM	X-linked dilated cardiomyopathy

Chapter 1

Introduction

Duchenne muscular dystrophy (DMD) is the second most common single gene disorder in Western countries and has been recognized as a distinct entity for over 100 years. In the last 40 years or so it has generated a great deal of interest among research workers and, in their bibliography of what they considered to be the more important publications on the subject up to 1985, Herrmann and Spiegler (1985) listed no fewer than 789 references. Yet, despite all the interest, the cause remained elusive until 1987. This was in part due to the fact that the tissue that is predominantly affected, namely, skeletal muscle, is complex as must also be the genetic repertoire responsible for its normal development and functioning.

There are 434 different muscles in the human body, which in the adult contribute to over 40 per cent of the total body weight. Much has been written on the development and morphology of muscle, but here only some general principles need be emphasized. The essential element of muscle is the muscle fibre (myofibre), which has been defined as '. . . a multinucleated cell that contains a large number of myofibrils embedded in a matrix of undifferentiated protoplasm, all enclosed within a fine sheath, the sarcolemma'. Muscle fibres are grouped together into fascicles and a network of collagen fibres surrounds each fascicle (perimysium), and extends between individual muscle fibres (endomysium). Each of the muscle fibres, which vary in length from one muscle to another, is bounded by the plasma membrane (plasmalemma) and an outer basement membrane (basal lamina). The latter along with the endomysium constitute the sarcolemma though this term is sometimes also used when referring to the plasma and basement membranes together (Fig. 1.1). Each multinucleated muscle fibre is formed during development by the fusion of several dividing mononucleated myoblasts derived from the myotomes. After fusion the nuclei of the fibre do not divide again and lie in the cytoplasm (sarcoplasm) along with the contractile elements. Small mononucleated satellite cells are situated between the plasma and basement membranes of the muscle fibre. These cells are believed to be a persistent population of myoblastic stem cells that retain the ability to divide and are a source of additional muscle

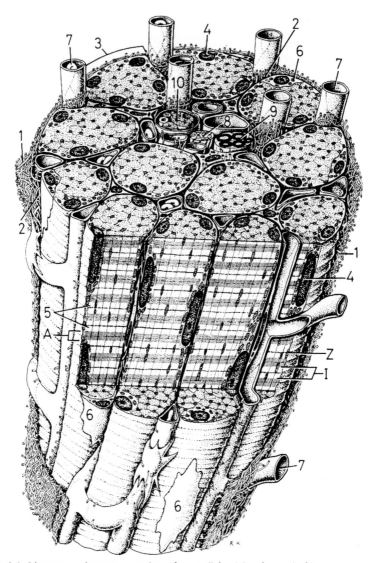

Fig. 1.1 Diagrammatic representation of a small fascicle of muscle fibres.
1, Perimysium; 2, endomysium; 3, muscle fibre (myofibre); 4, nucleus; 5, contractile
myofibrils; 6, satellite cells; 7, capillaries; A, dark bands; I, light bands; Z, Z-line.
(Reproduced from Krstič (1978) with kind permission of the author and publishers.)

fibre nuclei during growth and regenerative repair (Fig. 1.2). Recently, a population of pluripotent cells, distinct from satellite cells and named muscle-derived stem cells, was demonstrated in muscle.

A muscle fibre contains many myofibrils, which are the contractile elements of muscle and display alternating dark (A) and light (I) bands, and through

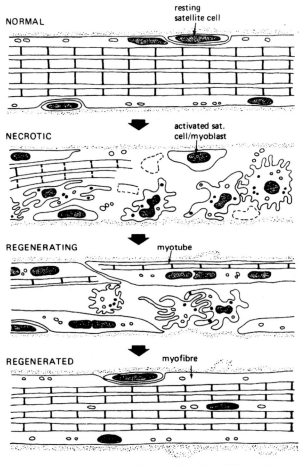

NORMAL

resting
satellite cell

NECROTIC

activated sat.
cell/myoblast

REGENERATING

myotube

REGENERATED

myofibre

Fig. 1.2 Diagrammatic representation of a satellite cell and its role in muscle fibre regeneration. (Reproduced by kind permission of Professor M.J. Cullen.)

the centre of the latter is the dense Z-line (band or disc) (see Fig. 1.1). The myofibrils are themselves composed of thick and thin myofilaments. During contraction and relaxation of the muscle, thin filaments slide between the thick filaments. In addition to nuclei and myofibrils, the sarcoplasm of a muscle fibre contains mitochondria, glycogen granules, lipid bodies, ribosomes, the transverse system of tubules (T-system), and the sarcoplasmic reticulum. The latter is equivalent to the endoplasmic reticulum of cells in other tissues and forms a network of tubules that run between the myofibrils. The T-system consists of transversely arranged, fine, interconnecting, tubular extensions of the plasma membrane. A single T-tubule and two dilated ends of the sarcoplasmic reticulum form so-called 'triads', which are concerned with the excitation and contraction of muscle fibres.

A nerve impulse, via the neuromuscular junction, produces depolarization of the muscle cell surface membrane, which then spreads inwards along the T-system to the triads. This results in the rapid release of calcium from the sarcoplasmic reticulum into the sarcoplasm, which in turn then results in the interaction between thick and thin filaments producing muscle contraction (Fig. 1.3).

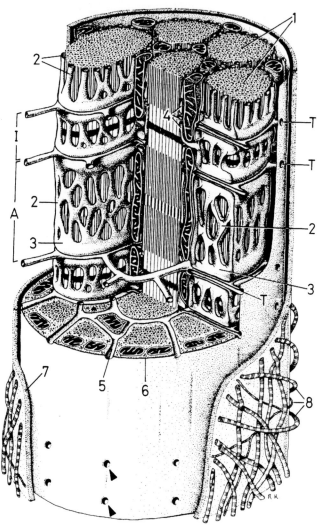

Fig. 1.3 Diagrammatic representation of a single muscle fibre. 1, Myofibril; 2 and 3, sarcoplasmic reticulum; T and 5, transverse tubular system; 4, triads; 6, plasma membrane; 7, basement membrane; 8, endomysium. (Reproduced from Krstič (1978) with kind permission of the author and publishers.)

Despite our increased understanding of the pathogenesis of DMD and Becker muscular dystrophy (BMD), we are still not certain about the mechanism of progressive muscle degeneration in these disorders. It is of interest to go through the mass of experimental information generated during the last decades on these dystrophies and compare it with our current knowledge about dystrophin and its localization and function. It is now clear that some of the data generated in the past are inconsistent with the current picture of this disease. However, some of the old data are intriguing and, during this edition of the book, we have referred quite extensively to this previous work wherever we felt it was of relevance.

During the process of selecting and emphasizing certain findings for the sake of clarity, it is inevitable that the resultant picture may be oversimplified, somewhat idiosyncratic, and probably inconsistent. The only defence is that voiced by Miguel de Unamuno in Erwin Schrödinger's (1944) book *What is life?*, which Watson and Crick and many others found so illuminating: 'If a man never contradicts himself, the reason must be that he virtually never says anything at all.'

A limited number of selected seminal references are quoted in each chapter, together with some of historical interest.

This book, which is partly based on cases and families studied by the authors, is not intended for the expert in any particular field, but rather for those with more catholic interests who are involved in this distressing and perplexing disease, which Gowers himself in 1879 referred to as being '. . . one of the most interesting and at the same time most sad'.

References

Gowers, W.R. (1879). *Pseudo-hypertrophic muscular paralysis—a clinical lecture.* J. and A. Churchill, London.

Herrmann, F.H. and Spiegler, A.W.J. (1985). *X-linked muscular dystrophies—a bibliography.* University Press, Leipzig.

Krstič, R.V. (1978). *Die Gewebe des Menschen und der Säugetiere.* Springer, Berlin.

Schrödinger, E. (1944). *What is life?* Cambridge University Press, Cambridge.

Chapter 2

History of the disease

Early beginnings

The history of the disease is an interesting one and was traced in detail in Emery and Emery (1995). Muscular dystrophy has no doubt afflicted humans from the earliest times. Since the ancient Egyptians in their wall paintings often depicted physical abnormalities with some care so that they can often be identified as diseases we now recognize, such as paralytic poliomyelitis and congenital dwarfism, it is just possible that they might have portrayed muscular dystrophy. In fact, it was suggested by the late Professor Becker that this might be so in a relief painting on the wall of a tomb in ancient Egypt, dating from the Eighteenth Dynasty of the New Kingdom, that is, about 1500 BC (Fig. 2.1). The subject depicted on the wall of the Temple of Hatshepsut is the Queen of Punt who shows lumbar lordosis and who, it has even been suggested, may also have some calf enlargement. However, in comparison with the adjoining figure she seems generally fatter, and perhaps what is shown is no more than generalized obesity.

However, on the wall of a tomb at Beni Hasan (illustrated in manuscripts at the Ashmolean Museum, Oxford), dating from the Middle Kingdom (circa 2800–2500 BC), one of us noticed that there are depicted two figures of interest (Fig. 2.2). The first has bilateral club foot. In the middle, however, is a boy with what could just possibly be muscular dystrophy. He has lost the normal arch of his feet, which is usually clear in Egyptian wall paintings as seen in the figure to the right. Also, his calves seem somewhat enlarged, and he may have some degree of (pseudo)hypertrophy of certain upper limb muscles. On the other hand, as the hieroglyph above his head implies, he may have been a dwarf.

The *Transfiguration* was Raphael's last great work, and was unfinished when he died on Good Friday, 1520, at the untimely age of 37. Vasari (1568), in his *Lives of the artists*, considers the boy in the painting to be 'possessed by a devil', an idea that may have prompted subsequent observers to suggest that it could illustrate a case of epilepsy. However, Duchenne himself, after whom the most common form of muscular dystrophy is named, when visiting the National

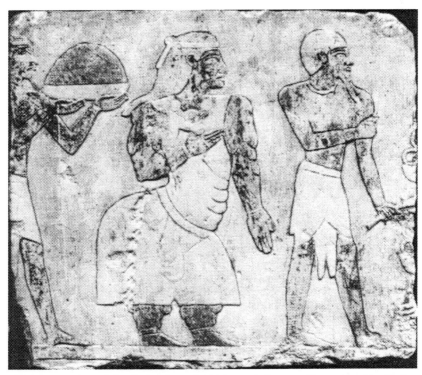

Fig. 2.1 Egyptian relief painting from the Eighteenth Dynasty. (Reproduced by kind permission of Professor P.E. Becker.)

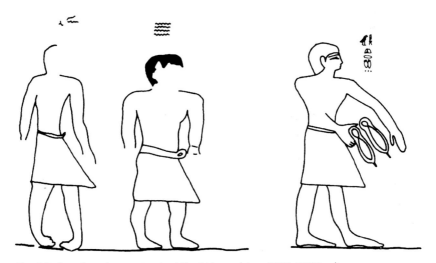

Fig. 2.2 Drawings from a tomb at Beni Hasan (circa 2800–2500 BC).

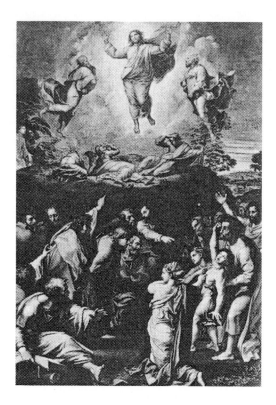

Fig. 2.3 Raphael's
Transfiguration.
(Reproduced by kind
permission of the Musei
Vaticani.)

Hospital for Nervous Diseases in London where a reproduction of the painting hung, commented at the time that the boy depicted by the artist might be
suffering from pseudohypertrophic muscular dystrophy (Fig. 2.3).

It is also interesting to note that William Harvey (1578–1657) should be
remembered not only for his observations on the circulation of the blood but
also for his studies in neurology and the structure and function of muscles. He
showed, for example, that muscles can be distinguished by their structure,
according to whether they are primarily fleshy, tendinous, sinewy, or membran-
ous, as well as their action in causing movement.

However, the first clinical descriptions of dystrophy itself, at least in the
English language, can be attributed to Charles Bell. He was born in
Fountainbridge in Edinburgh in 1774, where he studied medicine and subsequently worked as a surgeon–anatomist, often illustrating his works with his
own carefully executed drawings. At the age of 30 years he moved to London
where he spent most of his working life, and was a founder of the Middlesex
Medical School. He returned to Edinburgh to the Chair of Surgery in 1835, and
died in 1842 from angina. He is best remembered for being the first to describe
paralysis of the facial nerve (Bell's palsy) and, with the French experimental

physiologist, François Magendie, for discovering the distinct functions of the posterior (sensory) and anterior (motor) nerve roots of the spinal cord (Fig. 2.4).

Among his numerous publications is *The nervous system of the human body*. In it he describes (Case 89) an 18-year-old man with wasting and weakness of the quadriceps muscles that had begun some 8 years previously and that

> . . . disabled him from rising; and it is now curious to observe how he will twist and jerk his body to throw himself upright from his seat. I use this expression, for it is a very different motion from that of rising from the chair. (Bell 1830, p. CLXIII)

There was no sensory loss. Without muscle pathology the diagnosis cannot be certain, but the description would certainly be compatible with muscular dystrophy.

Gowers (1879), whose seminal contributions to the subject will be dealt with in more detail later, refers to the possibility of the disease having been described in 1838 by Coste and Gioja in the *Annali Clinici dell'Ospedale degli Incurabili di Napoli* which was abstracted in Schmidt's *Jahrbücher*. But this was a mistake. Recent research by Professor Giovanni Nigro of the University of Naples (Nigro 1986) has revealed that the cases in question were presented by Professor Gaetano Conte (*not* Coste) with the help of a Dr L. Gioja and reported in the journal in fact in 1836. Two brothers apparently first manifested the disease at age 8, had enlarged calves and progressive muscle wasting and weakness, which particularly affected the lower limbs, and subsequently developed contractures of the knees and hips. The elder brother died of cardiac failure. Sensory functions were intact and mentation was normal. The clinical features are presented in detail and the original publication has now been reproduced in full in *Cardiomyology* (Vol. V (No. 1) 1986, pp. 1–30).

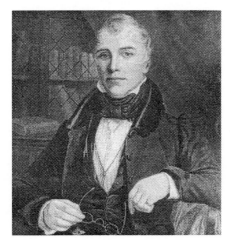

Fig. 2.4 Sir Charles Bell. (Reproduced by kind permission of the National Galleries of Scotland, Edinburgh.)

It seems very likely that these two brothers probably had muscular dystrophy though there is no report of muscle pathology. But certainly Professor Gaetano Conte, who was born in Naples in 1798 and dedicated most of his life to the study of 'scrofole' (?dystrophy), must rank among the pioneers in the history of the subject.

However, in 1847 a Mr Partridge presented a case to the Pathological Society of London (reported in the *London Medical Gazette* Vol. 5, p. 944) of a boy who, from about the age of 9 years, had developed progressive muscle wasting and weakness, had enlarged calves and muscle contractures, and who died after an attack of measles at age 14. Examination of muscle tissue at autopsy revealed widespread fatty degeneration. In the same year, 1847, Dr W.J. Little, a physician at the London Hospital, studied two affected brothers aged 12 and 14 whom he reported in detail in 1853 in a book entitled *On the nature and treatment of the deformities of the human frame*. Both brothers presented a similar picture. Onset was in early childhood with a tendency to walk on the toes and a peculiar gait with the '. . . head and body having been inclined backwards'. There was progressive muscle wasting and weakness affecting the neck, trunk, and upper and lower extremities associated with enlargement of the calf muscles and contractures 'behind the heels'. Sensation was normal. Both boys were unable to walk by the age of 11. The elder died at 14 and, at autopsy, examination of the gastrocnemius and soleus muscles (and some other muscles as well) revealed that the muscle tissue had been largely replaced by fat ('adipose degeneration'). The brain and spinal cord appeared normal. These findings would certainly be consistent with the diagnosis of the severe form of muscular dystrophy that predominantly affects boys. However, the fullest and earliest description of this disorder must clearly be credited to Dr Edward Meryon of St. Thomas's Hospital, London (Fig. 2.5).

Edward Meryon

Edward Meryon was born in 1809 and studied medicine in Paris and University College, London. He qualified as a Member of the Royal College of Surgeons in 1831, proceeding to an MD degree in 1844. His chief appointments were at St. Thomas's Hospital and the Hospital for Nervous Diseases where it is just possible he may have been acquainted with the young William Gowers. He was apparently a man of wide learning and published several books relating to the nervous system. He also embarked on a *History of medicine* but unfortunately did not get beyond a first volume. In Feiling's (1958) *History of the Maida Vale Hospital* the only reference to him reads: 'Edward Meryon although not really distinguished in medicine, was clearly a well-known figure in London society

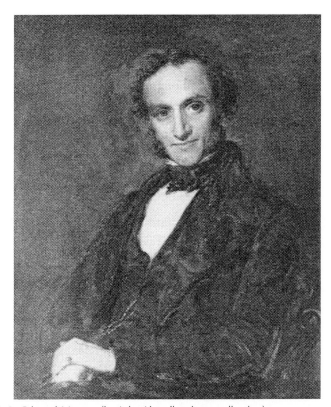

Fig. 2.5 Dr Edward Meryon (by John Linnell, private collection).

at the time'. He died at his home in Mayfair in 1880, at the age of 71 (Emery and Emery 1995).

In a communication addressed to the Royal Medical and Chirurgical Society in December 1851 and published in the Transactions of the Society the following year, Meryon described eight affected boys in three families. Interestingly, one of the two affected brothers in the second family is the case on which Partridge had earlier reported his autopsy findings in 1847. Meryon was particularly impressed by the familial nature of the condition and its predilection for males, and in his book, *Practical and pathological researches on the various forms of paralysis*, published in 1864, he details a family in which there were four affected cousins with the disorder having been transmitted through three sisters. Secondly, he subjected muscle tissue to microscopic examination and reported that

> . . . the striped elementary primitive fibres were found to be completely destroyed, the sarcous element being diffused, and in many places converted into oil globules and

granular matter, whilst the sarcolemma and tunic of the elementary fibre was broken down and destroyed. (Meryon 1852, p. 76)

He therefore used the term 'granular degeneration' for the microscopic changes he observed. Furthermore, his emphasis on the subsacolemma being broken down was certainly prescient. Some 130 years later the protein defect was shown to reside in the sarcolemma! Thirdly, he observed that

... the relative proportion of the grey matter to the white in the cord, and the ganglionic cells of the former, and the tubular structure of the latter, as well as of the nerves and the white substance within the neurolemma, wherever examined by the microscope, all bore evidence of the healthy condition of the nervous system. (Meryon 1852, p. 78)

Thus, he concluded that this was a familial disease with a predilection for males, which primarily affected muscle tissue and was not a disease of the nervous system. Meryon's clear delineation of the disorder and his understanding of its nature were very significant contributions. It is therefore unfortunate that he has not always been given the credit he deserves and that his work is completely overshadowed by that of Duchenne.

Duchenne de Boulogne

Guillaume Benjamin Amand Duchenne, Duchenne de Boulogne as he signed himself in order not to be confused with Duchesne of Paris, was born in the town of Boulogne-sur-Mer on 17 September 1806 (Fig. 2.6). He studied medicine in Paris where his teachers included Cruveilhier, Dupuytren, and Laennec. He then returned to Boulogne with the intention of being a family

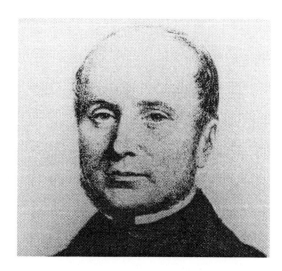

Fig. 2.6 Duchenne de Boulogne. (Reproduced from Haymaker (1953) courtesy of Charles C. Thomas, Springfield, Illinois.)

doctor. However, this proved a very unhappy time, for his young wife died of puerperal sepsis 14 days after giving birth to their son Emile in 1833, and for several years afterwards he remained depressed and lost interest in his work.

In 1839 he remarried, this time to a widow, but this does not seem to have been a happy marriage. Then in 1842, at the age of 36, he returned to Paris where he spent the rest of his life. It has been suggested there may have been three factors instrumental in his return to Paris and to neurology: his growing interest in the possible therapeutic effects of electricity; his own family history of a 'nervous' disease; and his disastrous second marriage. Whatever the reasons he quickly settled in Paris where he became a sort of itinerant physician mainly at the Salpêtrière. He never held an official hospital or academic appointment and was therefore completely free to pursue his obsessional interests in the electrical stimulation of muscle, muscle function, and neuromuscular diseases. He studied the mechanisms of facial expression, a subject that had also interested Charles Bell some years previously. His painstaking observations led to clear descriptions of several disorders, his name now being most closely associated with progressive muscular atrophy (with Aran) and progressive bulbar palsy (both part of the motor neuron disease complex), and of course pseudohypertrophic muscular dystrophy. He devised a strength gauge or dynamometer and a special needle-harpoon for muscle biopsy. The last 5 years of his life saw him famous but tragic: his wife died in 1870 and his son shortly afterwards from typhoid fever. He suffered a cerebral haemorrhage in August 1875, and Potain and Charcot never left him during the last weeks of his illness, taking it in turns to sleep by his bed. He died on 17 September 1875 on his 69th birthday. On 30 October the Paris correspondent of the *Lancet* (see Appendix A), commenting on Duchenne's life and work, wrote that, despite many adverse circumstances,

> ... his reputation has come out clear and bright as an honest, hard-working, acute, and ingenious observer, an original discoverer, a skilful professional man, and a kind-hearted, benevolent gentleman.

Despite his abounding interest in research, it seems he never lost a bedside manner.

Duchenne's interest in muscular dystrophy was first aroused in 1858 when his attention was drawn to a case, details of which he published in 1861 in the second edition of his book *De l'électrisation localisée* (Duchenne 1861). Later, in 1868, he reviewed in considerable detail his original case plus 12 further cases, two of whom were young girls, and referred to a further 15 cases in the German literature (Duchenne 1868). By 1870 he had seen some 40 cases of the disease, not counting those he saw when he visited the London hospitals around this time (Fig. 2.7).

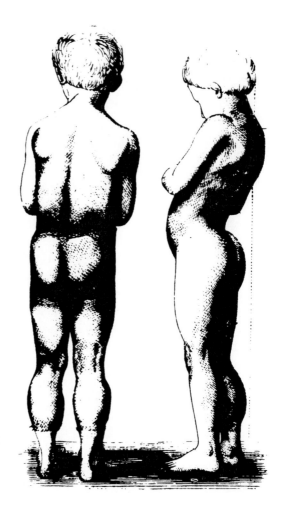

Fig. 2.7 Duchenne's original case, showing marked calf enlargement and lumbar lordosis. (From Duchenne (1868, p. 8).)

Duchenne defined the disease as being characterized by: progressive weakness of movement, first affecting the lower limbs and then later the upper limbs; a gradual increase in the size of many affected muscles; an increase in interstitial connective tissue in affected muscles with the production of abundant fibrous and adipose tissue in the later stages.

Though Meryon had studied the histology of affected muscles, his observations had been limited to material obtained at autopsy. Duchenne, on the other hand, used his needle-harpoon (*enporte-piéce histologique*) to obtain biopsy specimens in life. In fact, using this technique, he was able to study material from the same patient at different stages of the disease. His observations led him to conclude that the fundamental anatomical lesion was hyperplasia of the interstitial connective tissue which therefore prompted him to use the term *paralysie myosclérosique* as an alternative to *paralysie musculaire pseudohypertrophique*. Previously, a pathological diagnosis could only be made at autopsy, the so-called diagnosis of Morgagni. But Duchenne's technique meant that such a diagnosis could be made in life. He believed, correctly, that, unlike progressive (spinal) muscular atrophy of childhood, the disease was not caused by a lesion in the spinal cord. In this matter it is rather disappointing that Duchenne felt he should dismiss Meryon's contributions when he says that the latter confused the disease with progressive muscular atrophy, and therefore thought it had a neurogenic basis, which as we have seen he did not, and Duchenne goes further by giving the date of Meryon's address to the Royal Medical and Chirurgical Society as 1866 when in fact it was some 15 years earlier in 1851. Duchenne carefully weighed the available evidence regarding the possible aetiology of the disorder, particularly with regard to possible neurological or vasomotor factors, but had to conclude, just as we would have done until relatively recently, '. . . la pathogénie de la paralysie pseudo-hypertrophique est trés obscure; elle doit être réservée. . . .'

Though as we have seen Meryon had made a special note of his observation that the sarcolemma was broken down, a singularly important point, we now know that the primary defect does in fact reside in the sarcolemma.

William R. Gowers

Considerable interest now began to be shown in the disease and numerous case reports appeared in the French, English, German, American, Australian, and Danish literature. However, the next physician to enter the stage who made a significant contribution to the subject was William R. Gowers. Gowers was born in 1845 and spent all his life in London. He had a brilliant undergraduate career at University College Hospital where he was awarded medals in almost every subject of the medical curriculum and graduated with first class honours. He later became Professor of Medicine at University College, as well as being a physician at the National Hospital for Nervous Diseases. He was a man of immense intellect and wide interests. He was a knowledgeable botanist and an authority on mosses, an accomplished artist (he exhibited at the Royal Academy), and an obsessional shorthand writer. He introduced into medicine a number of new terms such as 'knee jerk', 'fibrositis', and 'abiotrophy'. He described several clinical signs including the nasal smile in myasthenia gravis, as well as the so-called Gowers' manoeuvre. He also invented a haemocytometer that was widely used for many years. It is understandable that in his day he was therefore widely admired and respected. He remained, however, a

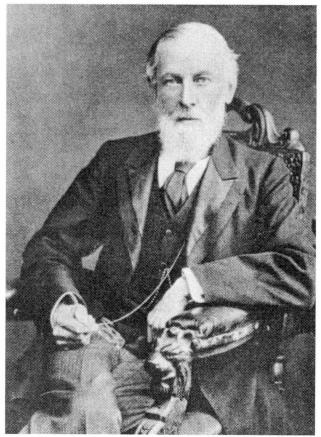

Fig. 2.8 Sir William Gowers. (Reproduced by kind permission of Dr Macdonald Critchley.)

reserved and very private individual with few intimate friends. He died in 1915 at the age of 70 (Fig. 2.8).

Gowers' interest in muscular dystrophy was kindled when working as a pre-medical student apprentice to a Dr Thomas Simpson in Coggeshall, Essex. Here he came across a family with four brothers afflicted with a 'strange disorder of locomotion with wasting of some muscles and enlargement of others'. Later he learned that the disease had been described in 1852 by Meryon and in 1879 he delivered a series of lectures on the disorder at the National Hospital which were published in *Lancet* and subsequently made into a monograph (Gowers 1879). The latter was based on information from 220 cases, which included 24 he had seen himself, 20 seen by colleagues, and the remainder from the literature. In deference to Duchenne he referred to the disease as 'pseudohypertrophic muscular paralysis', and in his monograph he attempted to give as complete a picture of the disease as possible with detailed discussions of the clinical features, pathology, prognosis, and possible treatment. As with all of Gowers' writings, clarity, thoughtfulness, and good prose are evident. This is illustrated in the graphic opening paragraph (Gowers 1879):

> The disease is one of the most interesting and at the same time most sad, of all those with which we have to deal: interesting on account of its peculiar features and mysterious nature; sad on account of our powerlessness to influence its course, except in a very slight degree, and on account of the conditions in which it occurs. It is a disease of early life and of early growth. Manifesting itself commonly at the transition from infancy to childhood, it develops with the child's development, grows with his growth—so that every increase in stature means an increase in weakness, and each year takes him a step further on the road to a helpless infirmity, and in most cases to an early and inevitable death.

The interest in the book lies mainly in the detailed presentation of the clinical features of the disease, and describes what is nowadays usually referred to as Gowers' manoeuvre or Gowers' sign (Fig. 2.9). Weakness of the hip and knee extensors causes difficulty in rising from the floor or a chair. As a result, when getting up, patients

> ... first put the hands on the ground (1), then stretch out the legs behind them far apart, and, the chief weight of the trunk resting on the hands, by keeping the toes on the ground and pushing the body backwards, they manage to get the knees extended so that the trunk is supported by the hands and feet, all placed as widely apart as possible (2). Next the hands are moved alternately along the ground backwards so as to bring a larger portion of the weight of the trunk over the legs. Then one hand is placed upon the knee (3), and a push with this and with the other hand on the ground is sufficient to enable the extensors of the hip to bring the trunk into the upright posture.

Gowers recognized that this had also been noted by Duchenne: 'If he bent forward he could only recover his position by catching hold of the furniture, or by supporting his hands on his thighs'. At first, Gowers thought the action of putting the hands on the knees, then grasping the thighs higher and higher ('climbing up his thighs') so as to extend the hips and push up the trunk was pathognomonic for the disease. However, he later realized that it could also be seen in other diseases in which the same muscle groups were affected.

Gowers also emphasized that the disease was primarily a disease of muscle and that the spinal cord was unaffected. Further, he was impressed by the predilection for males and was clearly convinced of the hereditary nature of the disorder. Of the total of 220 cases only 30 were females and these were usually less severely affected. Although isolated cases were common, he was impressed by the frequency with which other relatives could be affected (of the 220 cases,

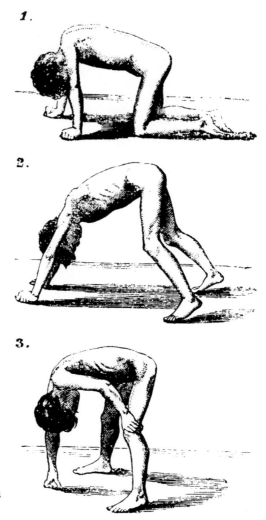

Fig. 2.9 Gowers' sign or manoeuvre. (From Gowers (1879).)

102 were isolated and 118 were grouped in 39 families). Perhaps his most revealing observation was that '. . . the disease is almost never to be heard of on the side of the father; when antecedent cases have occurred they have almost invariably been on the side of the mother'. Gowers also observed that a woman could have affected sons by different husbands, but found no instance in which members of the father's family suffered from the disease. He concluded that limitation to males and inheritance only through the mother was the same as in haemophilia. This pattern of inheritance was already recognized at the time,

although, in fact, it had been appreciated since the days of the *Talmud* some 1500 years earlier. The Jews excused from circumcision the sons of all the sisters of a mother who had a son with the 'bleeding disease'. The sons of the father's sibs were not so excused. The genetic basis for this mode of inheritance was appreciated through the rediscovery of Mendelism in 1900 and its cytological basis (X-linkage) recognized a few years later.

Wilhelm Heinrich Erb

By this stage in the story it was now quite clear that the disease primarily affected skeletal muscle and was hereditary. However, it was also clear that not all cases presented with exactly the same clinical features: females were occasionally affected and sometimes the disease in males would pursue a more benign course with survival into at least the third decade (for example, Gowers' cases 23, 35, and 36). This raised the possibility that perhaps after all there was more than one disease, an idea first pursued by Erb.

Wilhelm Heinrich Erb (Fig. 2.10) was born in 1840 in Bavaria and studied medicine at Heidelberg, Erlangen, and Munich. His subsequent professional life was spent almost entirely in Heidelberg. Erb was without doubt one of the greatest clinical neurologists of all time (Kuhn and Rüdel 1990). But he was also a great clinical teacher—the archetype of the time: severe, cultured, and always impeccably dressed. He died of a heart attack when he was 81—it is said whilst listening to Beethoven's *Eroica*.

Erb was greatly influenced by the studies of Duchenne, both with regard to the possible diagnostic and therapeutic uses of electricity in neurology, as well as his work on muscle disease. His pathological studies convinced him that the disease was due to a degeneration of muscle tissue and he coined the term 'Dystrophia muscularis progressiva' or progressive muscular dystrophy, a term that has been used ever since (Erb 1884). Many of the cases he studied were clearly different from cases described by Duchenne and he was well aware of this. In fact, he is credited with being the first to attempt to classify this group of diseases (Erb 1891). The details of his classification would now be questioned, but the idea that this was not one disease but a heterogeneous group of disorders was certainly true.

Recognition of heterogeneity

Over the next few decades, as physicians began to study their patients in increasing detail, attempts began to be made to categorize different types and to classify them according to various clinical criteria, such as distribution of

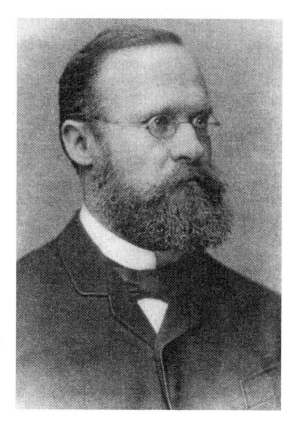

Fig. 2.10 Wilhelm Heinrich Erb. (Reproduced from Haymaker (1953) courtesy of Charles C. Thomas, Springfield, Illinois.)

muscle weakness and age at onset and progression. Later, the mode of inheritance was added. Although there were a few who continued for a while to believe that muscular dystrophy was essentially one disease, this view was gradually abandoned. However, there is a serious problem in considering heterogeneity within a group of disorders such as the muscular dystrophies. Differences between disease entities may be more apparent than real—variations within a spectrum and not necessarily a reflection of true genetic differences. This is constantly to be borne in mind when attempting to resolve apparent heterogeneity. The sentiments of Francis Bacon in 1620 are therefore apt:

> The steady and acute mind can fix its contemplations and dwell and fasten on the subtlest distinctions: the lofty and discursive mind recognises and puts together the finest and most general resemblances. Both kinds however easily err in excess, by catching the one at gradations the other at shadows.

How heterogeneity within this group of diseases was gradually resolved makes a fascinating byway in the history of medicine. However, there would be little value here in summarizing the detailed findings of these earlier studies,

Table 2.1 Clinical, biochemical, and genetic classification of the muscular dystrophies due to known gene defects

1	**Protein of the extracellular matrix**
	Collagen VI (Ullrich congenital muscular dystrophy)
	Laminin α2 (merosin-deficient congenital muscular dystrophy)
2	**Transarcolemmal proteins**
	Dystrophin (Duchenne and Becker muscular dystrophies/X-linked dilated cardiomyopathy)
	α sarcoglycan (severe childhood onset autosomal recessive muscular dystrophy (SCARMD) or limb girdle muscular dystrophy (LGMD)2D)
	β sarcoglycan (SCARMD or LGMD2E)
	γ sarcoglycan (SCARMD or LGMD2C)
	δ sarcoglycan (SCARMD or LGMD2F)
	Dysferlin (LGMD2B/Miyoshi myopathy)
	Caveolin (LGMD1C)
	Integrin α7 (congenital myopathy/dystrophy)
3	**Nuclear proteins**
	Emerin (X-linked Emery–Dreifuss muscular dystrophy)
	Lamin A/C (Autosomal dominant and autosomal recessive Emery–Dreifuss muscular dystrophy/dilated cardiomyopathy with conduction system disease)
	poly A binding protein 2 (PABP2) (oculopharyngeal muscular dystrophy)
4	**Sarcomeric proteins**
	Myotilin (LGMD1A)
	Telethonin (LGMD2G)
5	**Proteins with enzymatic activity**
	Calpain 3 (LGMD2A)
	Fukutin (Fukuyama congenital muscular dystrophy)
	FKRP (congenital muscular dystrophy MDC1C; LGMD2I)
	POMGnT1 (muscle–eye–brain disease)
	POMT1 (Walker Warburg syndrome)
	TRIM32 (LGMD2H)

which in any event have been critically reviewed elsewhere (Emery and Emery 1995). A classification based on current information favoured by the authors is reproduced in Table 2.1.

At this point perhaps it would be appropriate to consider which disorders are included under the heading 'muscular dystrophies'. For practical purposes a useful definition is 'a group of inherited disorders that are characterized by a progressive muscle wasting and weakness, in which the muscle histology has certain distinctive features (muscle fibre necrosis, phagocytosis, fibrosis, etc.) and where there is no clinical or laboratory evidence of spinal cord or peripheral nervous system involvement or myotonia'. Excluded, therefore, are the myotonic syndromes and the various congenital myopathies. However, such a definition encompasses disorders that vary considerably in their onset, severity, and distribution of muscle involvement. At one extreme there is the rapidly progressive form of congenital muscular dystrophy, which is present at birth with generalized muscle involvement. At the other extreme there is ocular muscular dystrophy where onset is in adult life and the disease is often limited to the extra-ocular muscles and may be no more than a minor inconvenience.

In this book we shall concentrate on that form of dystrophy associated with the name of Duchenne. Until fairly recently eponyms were retained for several other related forms of dystrophy such as the scapulohumeral (Erb), pelvifemoral (Leyden—Möbius), and the facioscapulohumeral (Landouzy–Dejerine) forms. But this habit has now been largely abandoned in favour of a clinical–genetic nomenclature. However, there remains one important exception; the retention of Becker's name for the X-linked form of the disease that clinically resembles Duchenne muscular dystrophy but is more benign with affected individuals often surviving into middle age.

Becker was, until his retirement in 1975, Professor of Human Genetics at the University of Göttingen, a position he had held since 1957. He died in 2001 (Fig. 2.11). Although by training a neurologist and psychiatrist, most of his work was centred on human genetics. The dystrophy that bears his name was first brought to his attention by Dr Franz Kiener, a psychologist in Regensburg, who sought Becker's advice on the disease that had affected several of his own

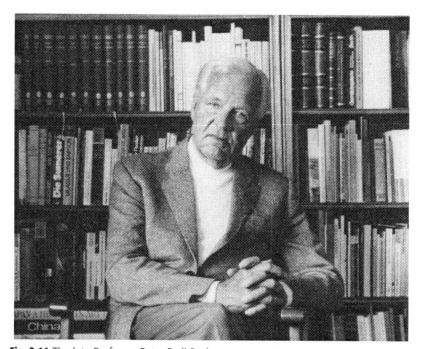

Fig. 2.11 The late Professor Peter Emil Becker.

relatives. Together, they studied the family in detail (Becker and Kiener 1955) and, a few years later, Becker reported two further families with the same disease (Becker 1962). Patients with the disease had been observed previously by others, but it was Becker who showed that it was clearly a separate clinical entity. It is now known that Duchenne and Becker types of muscular dystrophy are due to mutations at the same locus on the X chromosome. That is, they are allelic.

Recent developments

Some important landmarks in the history of Duchenne muscular dystrophy (DMD) are listed in Table 2.2. The recent history of DMD started in the late 1970s with the mapping of the defective gene to a specific locus on the short arm of the X chromosome (Xp2l). Within a few years gene-specific probes became available, culminating in the identification and characterization of the defective protein in Duchenne and Becker muscular dystrophies, namely, dystrophin. Many individuals have played important roles in these studies, the most notable being Dr Kay Davies of Oxford, Dr Lou Kunkel of Boston, Dr Ron Worton of Toronto, and Dr Eric Hoffman of Pittsburgh (Fig. 2.12). These developments will be discussed in detail in the text.

Table 2.2 Landmarks in the history of Duchenne muscular dystrophy (DMD)

Nineteenth century	DMD recognized as a specific clinical disorder (Conte and Gioja 1836; Meryon 1852; Duchenne 1861, 1868; Gowers 1879)
1955	Becker type muscular dystrophy (BMD) recognized as a distinct X-linked muscular dystrophy
1959–60	Serum creatine kinase (SCK) raised in patients and in female carriers
1978–83	DMD mapped to Xp2l by X/A translocations
1983–84	BMD and DMD shown to be allelic
1985	Gene-specific probes
1987–88	Gene deletions detected; cDNA cloned and sequenced Protein product (dystrophin) identified
1989–90	Dystrophin localization and functional studies begin Myoblast transfer experiments in mouse and humans First randomized controlled trials of glucocorticoids
1990–2	Gene transfer experiments in animal model
1992–4	Negative results of controlled studies on myoblast transfer in humans Identification of the dystrophin-like molecule, utrophin Identification of the dystrophin-associated glycoprotein complex
1999	Possibility of stem cell therapy in animal models

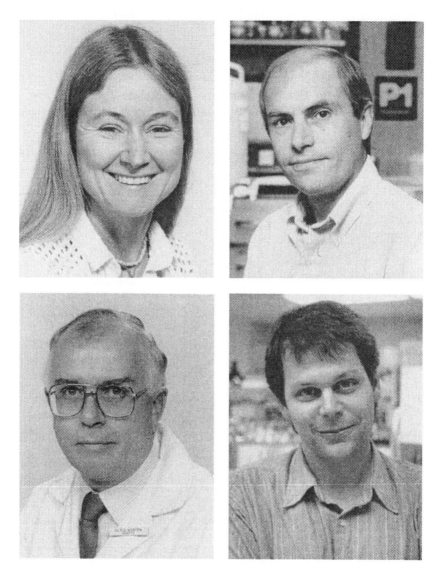

Fig. 2.12 Investigators who have played leading roles in recent research that has led to the localization and characterization of the Duchenne gene and its product. (Above) Drs Kay Davies and Lou Kunkel; (below) Drs Ron Worton and Eric Hoffman.

Based on these various findings rational new approaches to therapy are beginning to be considered. The prospects are now more hopeful than ever that, in the not too distant future, an effective therapy will be found for this tragic disease.

References

Becker, P.E. (1962). Two new families of benign sex-linked recessive muscular dystrophy. *Revue Canadienne de Biologie* **21**, 551–66.

Becker, P.E. and Kiener, F. (1955). Eine neue X-chromosomale Muskeldystrophie. *Archiv für Psychiatric und Nervenkrankheiten* **193**, 427–48.

Bell, C. (1830). *The nervous system of the human body: as explained in a series of papers read before the Royal Society of London.* Adam and Charles Black, Edinburgh.

Conte, G. and Gioja, L. (1836). Scrofola del sistema muscolare. *Annali clinic dell'Ospedale degli Incurabili di Napoli* **2**, 66–79.

Duchenne, G.B.A. (1861). *De l'electrisation localisee et son application a la pathologie et a la therapeutique,* 2nd edn. Baillière et fils, Paris.

Duchenne, G.B.A. (1868). Recherches sur la paralysie musculaire pseudohypertrophique ou paralysie myo-sclérosique. *Archives Génerales de Médecine* **11**, 5–25, 179–209, 305–321, 421–423, 552, 588.

Emery, A.E.H. and Emery, M. (1995). *The history of a genetic disease.* RSM Press, London.

Erb, W.H. (1884). Uber die 'juvenile Form' der progressiven Muskelatropie und ihre Beziehungen zur sogenannten Pseudohypertrophie del Muskeln. *Deutsches Archiv für Klinische Medizin* **34**, 467–519.

Erb, W.H. (1891). Dystrophia muscularis progressiva—klinische und pathologisch–anatomische Studien. *Deutsche Zeitschrift für Nervenheilkunde* **1**, 13–261.

Feiling, A. (1958). *A history of the Maida Vale Hospital for nervous diseases.* Butterworths, London.

Gowers, W.R. (1879). *Psuedo-hypertrophic muscular paralysis—a clinical lecture.* J. and A. Churchill, London.

Haymaker, W. (ed.) (1953). *The founders of neurology.* Charles C. Thomas, Springfield, Illinois.

Kuhn, E. and Rüdel, R. (1990). Wilhelm Heinrich Erb (1840–1921). *Muscle and Nerve* **13**, 567–9.

Little, W.J. (1853). *On the nature and treatment of the deformities of the human frame: being a course of lectures delivered at the Royal Orthopaedic Hospital in 1843,* pp. 14–16. Longman, Brown, Green, and Longmans, London.

Meryon, E. (1852). On granular and fatty degeneration of the voluntary muscles. *Medico-Chirurgical Transactions (London)* **35**, 73–84.

Meryon, E. (1864). *Practical and pathological researches on the various forms of paralysis.* Churchill, London.

Nigro, G. (1986). Conte or Duchenne? *Cardiomyology* **5**, 3–6.

Vasari, G. (1568). *Lives of the artists.* (Translated and printed by Penguin, London, 1981.)

Chapter 3

Clinical features

The skeletal muscle of children with Duchenne muscular dystrophy (DMD) can function quite well in the preclinical stages despite the presence of histological changes in the muscle biopsy. It is, however, more fragile compared to normal muscle and cannot sustain its physiological function without being damaged. The weakness only starts to appear when a significant part of skeletal muscle has degenerated and been replaced by fibro-adipose tissue. As a result of this the onset of clinical signs and symptoms is insidious and parents may be unaware that anything is wrong for some time.

Onset

Occasionally, mothers volunteer that their affected son seemed 'floppy' at birth and in infancy. However, this is never as pronounced or as frequent as in the congenital forms of muscular dystrophy or infantile spinal muscular atrophy (Werdnig–Hoffmann disease).

In a careful follow-up study some years ago of 109 infants presenting with hypotonia at birth or shortly after birth, 60 per cent were found to be affected by the severe form of spinal muscular atrophy (Werdnig–Hoffmann disease), 20 per cent by one of the congenital myopathies, and the remainder by a variety of conditions including cerebral palsy and mental handicap. Three of the 109 cases in the study went on to develop DMD. Also recently, rare cases of DMD with an early, infantile onset have been reported. However, the occurrence of this is exceptional, and is frequently associated with severe mental retardation.

The most common presentation is delay in walking and unsteady gait, with a tendency to walk on tiptoes. Of 114 cases in which this information was reliably documented, in 64 (56 per cent) walking was delayed until at least 18 months (Table 3.1) and roughly a quarter did not walk until they were at least 2 years old. In normal children, by comparison, the average age for learning to walk is about 13 months, and 97 per cent are walking by 18 months.

Approximate percentiles for age at apparent onset in 144 cases are given in Table 3.2. In this and other age-related events based on cases studied by one of the authors, percentiles were obtained by fitting the best curve to the data. It will be seen that in 90 per cent of cases onset is before school age (about

Table 3.1 Distribution of age at learning to walk in 114 affected boys

Age (months)	Number	Cumulative (%)
8–9	1	0.9
10–11	3	3.5
12–13	10	12.3
14–15	20	29.8
16–17	16	43.8
18–19	26	66.6
20–21	6	71.9
22–23	3	74.5
24–25	21	92.9
26–27	1	93.8
28–29	0	93.8
30–31	3	96.4
32–33	0	96.4
34–35	0	96.4
36	4	99.9

Table 3.2 Percentile distribution of age at apparent onset in 144 affected boys

Percentile	Age (years)
25	<2
50	2.4
60	2.8
70	3.4
75	3.7
80	4.1
90	5.1
95	6.1
99	7.8

5 years). Despite our increased understanding of DMD and the improved diagnostic tools, a recent survey published in 1999 by Bushby *et al.* in the *Lancet* suggested that the mean age at diagnosis for DMD in the UK is 4 years 10 months, virtually identical to the age at diagnosis in the early 1980s.

Table 3.3 Age at onset in affected brothers

Case number	Age at onset (years)		
	1st born	2nd born	3rd born
11	2	7	—
90	5	3	—
100	2.5	5	—
111	2.5	4	—
121	1.75	1.5	—
528	1.5	6	—
587	4	2.5	—
593	7.5	7.5	—
1761	4.5	4.5	4.5
2009	3	1.5	—

It is often stated that, if the parents have already had an affected son, the onset of the disorder in a second affected son is noted to be earlier because they are conscious of the possibility. But this is by no means always true as shown in Table 3.3 where age at onset is given for affected brothers in cases where this information was personally recorded by one of the authors *at the time the diagnosis was confirmed* in each case.

On close questioning in almost all cases, the affected child *was never able to run properly*. Other complaints at the time of onset included waddling gait, walking unsteadily with a tendency to fall easily, walking on toes, and difficulty in rising from the floor and climbing stairs. In a few instances weakness was first noticed after the child had sustained a fracture following a fall. Sometimes the parents noted a tendency to 'throw out his leg' when walking, for the 'feet to turn in', or their attention was even drawn to enlargement of the calf muscles (Fig. 3.1).

Although most cases present in early childhood, occasionally the diagnosis is not made until the age of 8 or 9. Even in these cases the classical difficulties of early childhood can always be elicited retrospectively. This is confirmed by several 'late' presenters assessed by one of the authors and reported in Table 3.4.

Other presenting features

The most common additional feature at presentation is delayed intellectual milestones and, in particular, delay in speech development. Some 50–70 per cent of DMD children will have a delay in speech at presentation. It is not

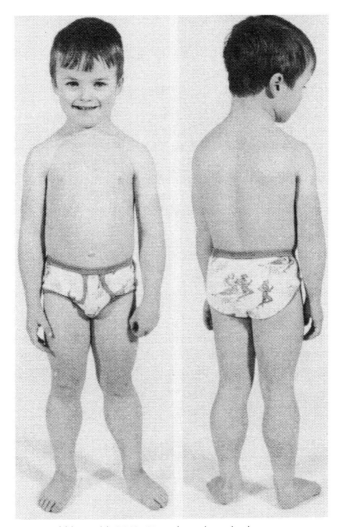

Fig. 3.1 A 4-year-old boy with DMD. Note the enlarged calves.

Table 3.4 Cases with delayed onset

Case number	Age (years)		Death	Comments
	Onset	Chairbound		
144	8	—	—	Now aged 10 and moderately affected
124	8	11	20	—
1741	8	12	—	Parents not good witnesses
2197	9	11	—	Severely mentally retarded (IQ < 50)
112	9	12	21	—

uncommon that concern related to the delay in speech precedes concerns related to the delayed motor development and muscle weakness. While the majority of children presenting with speech delay later on acquire the ability to speak normally, one-third of cases are eventually left with a significant delay. Autistic-like behaviour can on rare occasions be the presenting feature in some children with severe mental retardation (see below).

Muscle cramps are very rare and myoglobinuria following exercise is exceptional in DMD, but more common in Becker type muscular dystrophy (BMD). Often children with DMD complain of tenderness of their muscles after exercise.

'Failure to thrive' may, in some cases, be associated with the subsequent development of DMD. In keeping with previous observations, the authors have observed several children who presented in the first 18 months of life with unexplained failure to thrive. It is possible that this complication is secondary to the excessive muscle breakdown that is characteristic of these early phases of the disorder, although this remains speculative.

Because of these associations, it is suggested that any male infant who fails to thrive or where there is delay in motor, mental, or speech development for no apparent reason should have his serum creatine kinase level determined in order to exclude the possibility of DMD.

Muscle pseudohypertrophy

The most obvious feature in the early stages of the disease is enlargement of the calf muscles, which are often said to feel 'firm' or 'woody'. Of 89 cases where the size of the calves was noted at some time in the course of the disease, in at least 85 (96 per cent) they seemed much larger than normal. However, such enlargement may also involve the masseters, deltoids, serrati anterior, and quadriceps, and occasionally other muscles as well. Muscle enlargement is due, at least in part, to an excess of adipose and connective tissue, and therefore the term 'pseudohypertrophy' is widely used. But true (work) hypertrophy may also play a role as a compensation for weakness in other muscles. However, in DMD it is difficult to imagine this as being an important factor because in some cases such muscle enlargement can be extensive (Fig. 3.2). Enlargement of the tongue is a relatively frequent but late feature of the disease.

Interestingly, if in an affected boy a limb becomes affected by poliomyelitis, then there is no pseudohypertrophy in that limb and it therefore, presumably, depends on an intact nerve supply. Pseudohypertrophy is not pathognomonic for DMD since it can also occur in some other forms of dystrophy (typically in sarcoglycanopathies and limb girdle muscular dystrophy (LGMD)2I) and even occasionally in the mild form of spinal muscular atrophy.

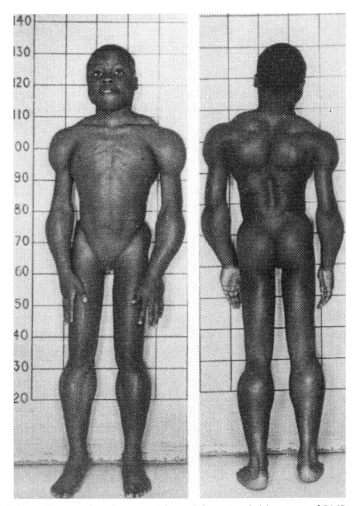

Fig. 3.2 Extensive muscle enlargement (pseudohypertrophy) in a case of DMD. (Reproduced by kind permission of Dr Sarah Bundey.)

Distribution of muscle weakness

Muscle involvement is always bilateral and symmetrical. In general, in the early stages of the disease the lower limbs are affected more than the upper limbs, and the proximal muscles more than the distal muscles. At this stage certain muscles are predominantly affected. These include the latissimus dorsi, sternocostal head of the pectoralis major, brachioradialis, biceps, triceps, iliopsoas, glutei, and quadriceps muscles. The involvement is highly selective. For example, the quadriceps are more affected than the hamstrings, triceps more than biceps, wrist extensors more than flexors, neck flexors more than extensors, dorsiflexors of the feet more than the plantar flexors. Even within a single muscle there is differential involvement. For example, the sternocostal head of the pectoralis major muscle is more affected than the clavicular head, but in contrast the clavicular head of the sternomastoid muscle is more affected than the sternal head. This differential muscle involvement becomes less clear as the disease progresses so that ultimately such patterns are no longer obvious. Later slight facial weakness often develops and the intercostal muscles also become affected. This can be followed by the involvement of the chewing and swallowing muscles. Sphincter control is never lost.

Early signs

This pattern of muscle involvement results in several well-defined physical features associated with the disease. Weakness of the gluteus medius and minimus muscles (which abduct the hip and hold the pelvic bone down to the greater trochanter of the femur) results in the pelvis tilting down toward the unsupported side when an affected child raises his leg from the ground (positive Trendeleburg sign). To compensate for this he inclines toward the supporting leg. As he moves forward this action is continually repeated and results in the broad-based, waddling gait that is so characteristic of DMD. But, as Professor Dubowitz (1995) has pointed out, 'not everything that waddles is muscular dystrophy' for other conditions can also produce this type of gait (for example, spinal muscular atrophy). Weakness of the gluteus maximus muscle (which powerfully extends the hip) results in a tendency for the pelvis to tilt forward and, in order to compensate for this, a lumbar lordosis develops. In order to maintain his balance, and possibly because of an imbalance between the dorsiflexors and plantar flexors, the affected child also tends to walk on his toes.

Weakness of the knee and hip extensors results in the classical Gowers' manoeuvre: the child climbs up his thighs in order to extend the hips and push up the trunk (Figs 2.9 and 3.3). However, it may be impossible to elicit this sign before the age of 4 or 5 years. Even before this age we have found that an affected child is unable to rise from a sitting position on the floor if he is asked to *keep his arms folded* (which prevents him from pushing on his thighs or on the floor), whereas a normal child can accomplish this quite easily.

In the early stages of the disease it may also be difficult to elicit weakness of the pectoral girdle musculature by formal testing. However, if the child is grasped around the chest from behind and an attempt made to lift him, there is a tendency to 'slide-through' the examiner's arms. Also, by placing the examiner's

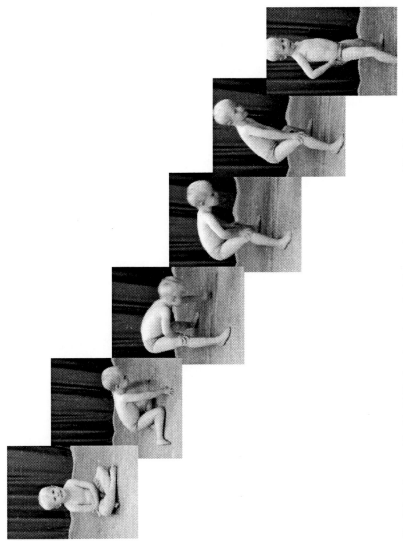

Fig. 3.3 A 5-year-old with DMD showing the typical Gowers' manoeuvre while rising from the floor.

hands inside the upper arms, a normal child can be held up with comparative ease, but not an affected child. Both these signs are positive by the age of 4 and sometimes earlier. As the disease progresses, winging of the scapulae becomes apparent.

The affected muscles are not tender (which could suggest oedema, a sign of myositis) and there is no voluntary or percussion myotonia. As the muscles become weaker and wasted, the corresponding tendon reflexes become depressed, though good ankle jerks are retained for a long time and are the last of the tendon reflexes to disappear. The plantar responses are always flexor and there is no sensory loss.

In the early stages of the disease, apart from the obvious difficulties of trying to keep up with their peers, affected boys usually make few complaints apart from occasionally tenderness and stiffness following exercise, particularly in the calf muscles.

Another frequent complaint is the walking on tiptoes, which becomes more evident when children are attempting to run or are tired. This is at least in part due to shortening of the heel cords (Achilles tendon). Most children with DMD have contractures of the Achilles tendon and more rarely of the hip flexors and ileotibial band or hamstrings at presentation.

Progression

The weakness is progressive but nevertheless often shows periods of apparent arrest. It is because of this fluctuation that the assessment of the efficacy of any suggested therapy has to be evaluated with considerable care.

As the disease progresses, the lumbar lordosis becomes more exaggerated and the waddling gait increases. Shortening of the Achilles tendon becomes more marked and an equinovarus deformity develops, though this is more obvious when the boy becomes confined to a wheelchair.

Respiratory muscles, although involved to some extent in all stages of the disorder, are never significantly weak in ambulant children, who will consistently have forced vital capacity (FVC) > 70 per cent before the child is wheelchair-dependent.

Although, initially, an affected boy may find he only needs a wheelchair at certain times (for example, when going outside), inevitably he will become permanently confined to a wheelchair. The age at which this occurs is more precise and much better documented than the age at onset (Table 3.5). In the series obtained by one of the authors and presented in this table, no attempts had been made to prolong ambulation by various orthopaedic measures and therefore the data relate to the natural progress of the disease.

Table 3.5 Percentile distribution of age at becoming confined to a wheelchair in 120 affected boys

Percentile	Age (years)
10	6.7
20	7.4
30	7.8
40	8.2
50	8.5
60	8.9
70	9.3
75	9.6
80	10.0
90	11.0
95	11.9
99	13.2

Of the 120 affected boys in which the age at becoming confined to a wheelchair was reliably known, in 95 per cent of cases this occurred by the age of 12. The age at becoming confined to a wheelchair was not significantly correlated with age at onset but was significantly correlated with age at death ($N = 55$; $r = 0.33$; $p < 0.02$). The difference in mean age at death in boys who became chairbound by 8 years of age ($N = 27$; mean, 16.23 years; standard deviation (SD), 2.66 years) compared with those who became chairbound after 8 years of age ($N = 28$; mean, 17.77 years; SD, 2.79 years) is statistically significant ($p < 0.05$). It would seem that age at death after 15 increases roughly by 1 year for each year that a boy remains ambulant after the age of 7 up to the age of 10 or more (Table 3.6). In general terms, the earlier a boy becomes confined to a wheelchair, the poorer the prognosis.

Assessment of motor ability

It is valuable to be able to chart the course of the disease in patients. A number of systems have been devised for doing this, which depend on assessing either muscle strength or functional ability.

1   Muscle strength
   - MRC grading (0–5)
   - Ergometry

Table 3.6 Age at death related to age at becoming confined to a wheelchair

	Age (years) confined to a wheelchair			
	≤7	8	9	10 or more
Number	9	18	15	13
Mean	15.65	16.52	17.44	18.15
SD	3.36	2.29	2.65	3.00
Number		27		28
Mean		16.23		17.77
SD		2.66		2.79

2   Functional ability

- Swinyard grade (1–8)
- Vignos grade (1–10)
- Hammersmith motor ability score (0–40)
- 'CIDD' grade for upper limbs (1–6)

Details of the various grading systems are given in Appendices B–F and will be discussed in more detail later. A very detailed functional scoring system has also been developed by Cornelio *et al.* (1982), which is expressed as the sum of single scores for gait, climbing stairs, getting up from a chair, and getting up from a seated position on the floor.

Since there is inevitably a subjective element in such methods, in order to make comparisons either between different patients or with the same patient over a period of time, they are best carried out by the same person. For many years one of the authors (A.E.) has used the Swinyard and Vignos grades of most patients examined (186 observations on 110 patients), and the results are given in Figs 3.4 and 3.5. Both grades correlate well with the progress of the disease. However, there is clearly considerable variation between different boys of the same age.

The other author (F.M.) has used the Hammersmith scale over the last 10 years in more than 200 children with DMD, monitored every 6 months. This scale can be easily administered in clinic or at the time of the physiotherapy assessment and is particularly useful for monitoring progression and effect of intervention in ambulant children. An example of the distribution of functional abilities in DMD children assessed with this scale is shown in Fig. 3.6. Control children acquire the ability to perform all the assigned tasks by the age of 4, while DMD children almost inevitably score <40/40 even in the early phases of the disease. Loss of independent ambulation usually occurs with

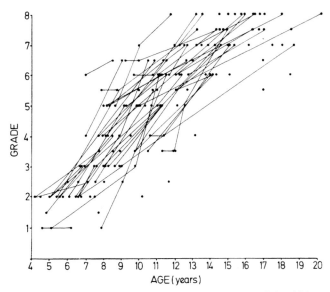

Fig. 3.4 Swinyard grade and age in boys with DMD. Points are joined for assessments on the same individual.

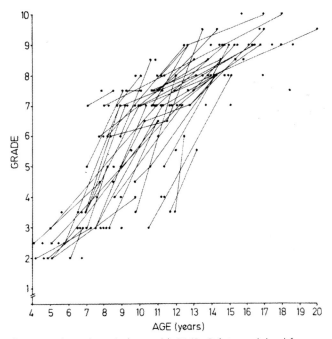

Fig. 3.5 Vignos grade and age in boys with DMD. Points are joined for assessments on the same individual.

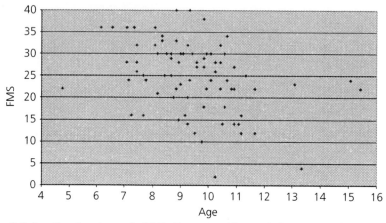

Fig. 3.6 Functional motor scale (FMS, Hammersmith Hospital motor scale) plotted against age in years in a cohort of children with DMD. Each point represent an assessment of a different child. The graph shows the progressive loss of function.

values ≤18/40. As this scale also highlights, there is a considerable spread of functional abilities for DMD children at any given age.

But, apart from variations in motor ability between boys of the same age, affected boys also differ in their general appearance. Some retain their subcutaneous fat and muscle bulk, whereas others become thin and atrophic. This is graphically demonstrated in the two boys of similar age shown in Fig. 3.7. The reason for this is not clear, but there is a tendency for affected brothers to follow a similar pattern. In most cases sexual development is normal though puberty is delayed in a proportion of cases.

Later stages

As the disease progresses and muscle weakness becomes more profound, contractures increasingly develop, particularly flexion contractures of the elbows, knees, hamstrings, and hips. Later, movements of the shoulders and wrists also become limited. Talipes equinovarus deformity becomes marked with the talus bone protruding prominently under the skin on the dorsum of the foot. Unless adequate support is provided in the wheelchair and, not infrequently despite the adequate support, a severe kyphoscoliosis develops. Thoracic deformity poses the most serious problem as it restricts adequate pulmonary airflow on the compressed side (Fig. 3.8).

The respiratory problems are also aggravated by weakness of the intercostal muscles. About halfway through the course of the disease a gradual deterioration begins in pulmonary function with reduced maximal inspiratory and

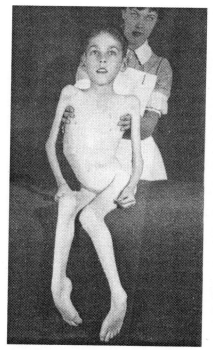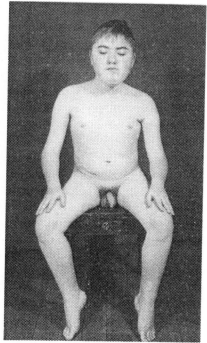

Fig. 3.7 A 13-year-old boy (left) and a 12-year-old boy (right) with DMD. (Reproduced from Dubowitz (1995) with the kind permission of the author and W.B. Saunders, the publishers.)

expiratory pressures. By the later stages there is a significant reduction in total lung capacity and an increase in residual volume.

While arterial oxygen tension (pO_2) and carbon dioxide tension (pCO_2) are normal both during the day and the night when children are ambulant, with the progressive decrease of respiratory function patients often slowly drift into respiratory failure. In DMD this usually does not occur when the FVC > 35 per cent, but is frequent for patients with FVC < 25 per cent. As the intercostal muscles are less used during the night, especially during deep sleep, the exclusive diaphragmatic breathing is not sufficient to maintain normal gas exchange during the night. The first sign of respiratory failure is therefore the night-time hypoventilation, with a fall in pO_2 and accumulation of carbon dioxide, followed by rapid restoration of normal gas tension following arousal. This 'early respiratory failure' phase can last for several months or even longer, but, when abnormal gas tensions also occur during the day, the prognosis for long-term survival is poor. Patients with diurnal hypercapnia will not survive more than 9.7 months (mean value) if respiratory assistance is not given.

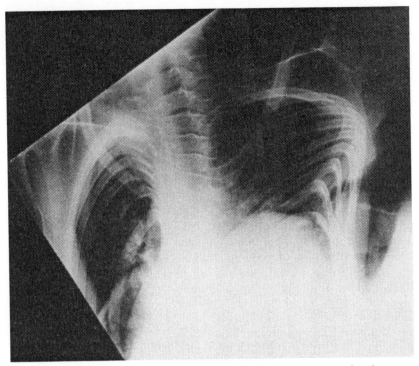

Fig. 3.8 Chest X-ray of an 18-year-old boy severely affected with DMD showing gross thoracic deformity.

More details on the intervention for night-time hypoventilation can be found in Chapter 13.

Cardiac muscle is also affected, as will be discussed later, but it is rare for a boy to succumb to heart failure though occasional cases of sudden death may be attributable to cardiac involvement.

In the personal experience of one of the authors, collected between 1965 and 1985, 14 cases of DMD came to autopsy and the primary causes of death were given as pneumonia (11), 'respiratory failure' (1), diphtheria at age 8 (1), and acute cardiac arrhythmia (1). Recent figures estimate that around 15 per cent of DMD cases will die of a primary cardiomyopathy.

That age at death might be in some way related to socio-economic factors is not borne out in the present series of patients. When information on social class was available there was no apparent relationship with age at death (Table 3.7).

Age at death was not significantly correlated with age at onset but, as we have seen, it was correlated with age at becoming confined to a wheelchair. The percentile distribution for DMD individuals of age at death in the year 1985 is given in Table 3.8. In 90 per cent of cases this occurred before the age of 20.

Table 3.7 Age at death in DMD and social class of parents

Age at death (years)	Number in social class[†]					
	5	4	3	2	1	Total
<10	—	1	—	—	1	1
10–14	1	1	4	2	—	8
15–19	4	15	11	5	1	36
20–24	2	—	1	—	—	3
Total	7	16	17	7	1	48

$$(\chi^2 = 10.92; p > 0.05)$$

[†] Social class is ranked from 5 (unskilled) to 1 (professional).

Table 3.8 Percentile distribution of age at death in 129 affected boys

Percentile	Age (years)
10	12.0
20	13.4
30	14.3
40	15.0
50	15.5
60	16.2
70	17.0
75	17.6
80	18.1
90	19.5
95	20.5
99	23.5

The considerable variation in the severity of the disease is further illustrated in Table 3.9 from which it can be seen that some boys may become chair-bound, or even die from the disease, before the apparent onset in other boys.

Recent data from Bushby suggests that intervention has changed the natural history of the disorder. While the mean age at death in the Northern region was 14.3 years in the 1960s, this improved to 19 years in the 1990s for non-ventilated patients. This is conceivably the result of the better management of these patients following the institution of the neuromuscular centre. This resulted, for example, in a better management of scoliosis and of intercurrent

Table 3.9 Numbers of boys with DMD with different ages at onset, becoming confined to a wheelchair, and death (author A.E.'s series up to 1985)

Age (years)	Number of boys with age at		
	Onset	Chairbound	Death
<2	24		
2	46		
3	27		
4	23		
5	14		
6	2	2	
7	3	15	
8	3	27	2
9	2	31	2
10		19	1
11		14	2
12		6	6
13		4	7
14		2	19
15			10
16			25
17			15
18			11
19			12
20			7
21			6
22			—
23			2
24			1
25			1
Total	144	120	129

respiratory infections. Following the recent introduction of assisted ventilation in the later stages of the disease (in the 1990s), the mean age of survival for those patients who do not develop early and severe cardiomyopathy has recently shifted to 24.3 years (Eagle *et al.* 2002; Fig. 3.9). This is well in keeping with our collaborative studies with Dr. Anita Simonds, indicating survival

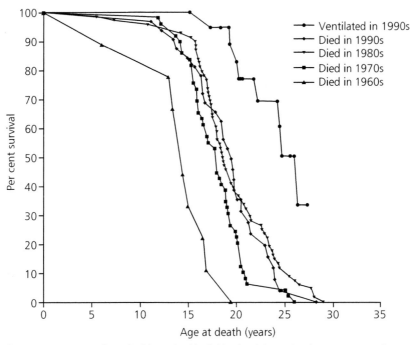

Fig. 3.9 Mean age of survival (years) of individuals with DMD. The mean age of survival for patients who do not develop an early and severe cardiomyopathy has recently shifted to over 26 years according to a recent study of Bushby in the UK northern region. (Reproduced with permission from Eagle *et al.* (2002).)

rates of 73 per cent after 5 years in ventilated DMD patients (Simonds *et al.* 1998) and includes patients who have been able to complete their university studies and one who had even fathered a child. The issue of assisted ventilation in DMD will be discussed in Chapter 13.

Disorders other than muscular dystrophy in affected boys

Several studies have shown that affected boys are of normal length and weight at birth but subsequently growth is slower than normal and later they are often of short stature. Otherwise, apart from mental handicap and problems directly relating to muscle weakness, most boys have very few health problems. The only other disorders recorded in the present series were recurrent urinary infections (2), left hydronephrosis with associated impaired renal function (1), unspecified congenital heart disease (1), undescended testes (1), and insulin-dependent diabetes mellitus (1). In the last case the same disease also affected the boy's father.

Children with DMD usually have larger head circumference compared to their healthy siblings. This may not be true for those children who carry mutations affecting the expression of Dp71.

Summary and conclusions

The onset of the disease is insidious but important hallmarks in the very early stages are frequent falls, tiptoe gait, and an inability to run properly. In over half the cases walking is delayed until at least 18 months of age. Manifestations of the disease are apparent in most cases before 5 years, but occasionally the diagnosis is delayed until the age of 8 or even 9 years of age. Many patients with the milder allelic variant Becker type muscular dystrophy (BMD) may also present in the first decade of life, with similar symptoms. There are a few useful clinical tips to help to differentiate DMD from BMD on clinical grounds. DMD children are not able to:

- run properly;
- hop on one leg;
- lift their head off the bed;
- get up from a sitting position on the floor if asked to keep their arms folded.

Conversely, children affected with BMD are typically able to run, hop, lift the head off the bed, and get up from the floor without a Gowers' manoeuvre, at least at presentation.

Pseudohypertrophy of the calf muscles is present in almost all cases of DMD and in some instances other muscles also show a pseudohypertrophic appearance. Wasting and weakness predominantly affects the proximal limb girdle musculature but early on muscle involvement is highly selective. A waddling gait, Gowers' sign, and 'sliding-through' the examiner's arms are useful diagnostic signs. However, even before Gowers' sign can be elicited, affected boys are unable to rise from a sitting position on the floor if asked to keep their arms folded. The age at becoming confined to a wheelchair (which is invariably before the 13th birthday) is a prognostic sign in that age at death after 15 increases roughly by 1 year for each year that a boy remains ambulant after the age of 7 up to the age of 10 or more.

While 90 per cent of boys died before the age of 20 until a decade ago, usually from respiratory problems, recent figures on ventilated individuals suggest that survival into the middle 20s can be achieved in a significant number of individuals. However, as with the other main events in the natural history of the disorder, there is considerable variation from one individual to another and early cardiac involvement is a negative prognostic factor.

References

Bushby, K.M., Hill, A., and Steele, J.G. (1999). Failure of early diagnosis in symptomatic Duchenne muscular dystrophy. *Lancet* **353** (9152), 557–8.

Cornelio, F., Dworzak, F., Morandi, L., Fedrizzi, E., Balsetrini, M.R., and Godoni, L. (1982). Functional evaluation of Duchenne muscular dystrophy: proposal for a protocol. *Italian Journal of Neurological Sciences* **4**, 323–30.

Dubowitz, V. (1995). *Muscle disorders in childhood.* W.B. Saunders, London.

Eagle, M., Baudouin, S.V., Chandler, C., Giddings, D.R., Bullock, R., and Bushby, K. (2002). Survival in Duchenne muscular dystrophy: improvements in life expectancy since 1967 and the impact of home nocturnal ventilation. *Neuromuscular Disorders* **12**, 926–9.

Simonds, A.K., Muntoni, F., Heather, S., and Fielding, S. (1998). Impact of nasal ventilation on survival in hypercapnic Duchenne muscular dystrophy. *Thorax* **53**, 949–52.

Chapter 4

Confirmation of the diagnosis

It is unlikely that an experienced physician would have any difficulty in suspecting Duchenne muscular dystrophy (DMD) in an otherwise healthy young boy who presents with a waddling gait, pseudohypertrophic calves, and a positive Gowers' sign. However, the diagnosis may not be so obvious in the very young or in those cases where onset is delayed until late childhood. Also, because of the uniformly poor prognosis and the parents' need for reliable genetic counselling, it is essential that the diagnosis be firmly established as soon as possible. This depends on:

1. careful clinical examination;
2. determination of serum creatine kinase;
3. muscle pathology;
4. genetic studies.

Serum creatine kinase

The enzyme creatine kinase (EC2.7.3.2) catalyses the reversible transfer of a phosphate group from creatine phosphate to adenosine diphosphate (ADP) forming creatine and adenosine triphosphate (ATP)

$$\text{Creatine phosphate} + \text{ADP} \leftrightarrow \text{Creatine} + \text{ATP}.$$

The International Union of Biochemistry suggested the systematic name ATP: creatine phosphotransferase with creatine kinase as the acceptable trivial name.

Over the years a number of methods have been developed for measuring the activity of the enzyme, each depending on one of three approaches, details of which can be found in the previous edition of the book.

In healthy infants in the immediate newborn period, the level of activity of serum creatine kinase (SCK) is often somewhat raised to around 200–300 international units (IU). This may be due to muscular anoxia or the result of physical trauma. But, within a few days of birth, levels fall to ones that are not very different from those of older children. In young boys there is no significant correlation with age, while in adolescence higher levels are not infrequent and may possibly be a reflection of increased muscle mass and physical activity at this period; otherwise, values are the same as in adults. The distribution of SCK levels in normal young healthy adult men is positively skewed with a few individuals having high levels. But most values in young healthy adult men are less than 200 IU, which is a little higher than in women, presumably because the latter have less muscle mass.

Sibley and Lehninger in 1949 were the first to note that a serum enzyme (in this case aldolase) could be raised in patients with muscular dystrophy. Some 10 years later Ebashi and his colleagues in Tokyo (Ebashi *et al.* 1959) also showed that creatine kinase activity is raised in the serum of patients with muscular dystrophy, and this was confirmed the following year by Dreyfus *et al.* (1960) in Paris. Even at birth and before the disease becomes clinically evident, SCK levels are considerably higher in boys with DMD than in normal boys—up to 100 times higher. However, as the disease progresses levels fall but only approach normal values in the very late stages of the disease (Fig. 4.1).

The most likely explanation for the very high SCK levels in DMD is that the enzyme originates in muscle and escapes into the serum. The much lower

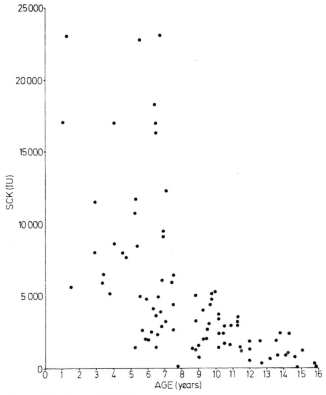

Fig. 4.1 SCK levels in boys with DMD.

levels in the later stages of the disease are no doubt due to the decrease in functioning muscle tissue and reduction in physical activity. Levels certainly decrease most around the time (age 8–10) when affected boys become confined to a wheelchair.

Grossly elevated SCK levels (50–100 times normal) occur not only in DMD but also in the early stages of Becker muscular dystrophy (BMD), in some of the limb-girdle muscular dystrophies (sarcoglycanopathies and limb girdle muscular dystrophies (LGMD) 2B and 2I), acute ischaemic muscle necrosis, and occasionally in the acute phase of polymyositis. Moderately elevated levels (up to 10 times normal) can occur in some other forms of muscular dystrophy (notably most of the limb girdle and facioscapulohumeral and a few congenital forms), mild spinal muscular atrophy, individuals predisposed to malignant hyperpyrexia, and occasionally in some other disorders including motor neuron disease, severe hypocalcaemia, and hypothyroidism. High SCK levels (MB isoform, see below) also occur with myocardial infarction. Thus, a boy with evidence of proximal muscle weakness, with a waddling gait, and a positive Gowers' sign, who is otherwise well and does not have polymyositis, but has a grossly elevated SCK level, is almost certainly suffering from DMD or BMD, as these conditions are far more common than the remaining dystrophies. Spontaneous myoglobinuria is rare but we have observed it in young children with DMD.

Creatine kinase isoenzymes

Creatine kinase (CK) exists in three molecular forms or isoenzymes. Each isoenzyme results from the dimeric association of two subunits referred to as M and B, and the three isoenzymes are designated as MM, MB, and BB. The BB isoenzyme predominates in brain tissue, whereas the MM isoenzyme predominates in cardiac and skeletal muscle. The hybrid MB isoenzyme is a minor component in both cardiac and skeletal muscle. In normal serum the isoenzyme is very largely MM with only about 4 per cent being MB. This small MB fraction, however, is significantly increased in patients with DMD or BMD. Though the MB form is found in cardiac muscle, its presence in serum in DMD is unrelated to cardiac involvement in the disease and presumably originates in dystrophic muscle in which there is more MB activity than in normal muscle. Bone also contains CK (BB isoenzyme). An increase in this isoenzyme has been reported in osteopetroses, bone tumours, and following fractures.

Other muscle enzymes that exist as isoenzymes and have been studied in detail in DMD are lactate dehydrogenase, aldolase, and pyruvate kinase. Lactate dehydrogenase (LDH) exists as five isoenzymes (LDH 1–5). In the serum of patients with DMD there is a relative increase in the proportions of LDH 1–3, which reflects changes in the isoenzyme pattern in affected muscle tissue. There are muscle, brain, and liver forms of aldolase and the serum activity in DMD is predominantly that of the muscle type. Pyruvate kinase (PK) exists as three isoenzymes (M2, M1, and L). In patients with DMD, serum activity is mainly of the M1 type, which is the only PK isoenzyme found in skeletal muscle and brain and the major component in cardiac muscle. Finally, carbonic anhydrase III and β-enolase are skeletal muscle-specific enzymes, and these too are elevated in the serum of affected boys. Thus, in all these instances the enzyme pattern in the serum of patients is similar to that in muscle tissue.

Other serum enzymes

Several other enzymes have been found to be raised in the serum in DMD, though none to the same extent as CK. The highest levels (10–20 times normal) occur with aldolase, pyruvate kinase, carbonic anhydrase III, and β-enolase. Less dramatic increases have been found in a number of other enzymes including:

- lactate dehydrogenase;
- phosphoglycerate mutase;
- alanine aminotransferase (glutamic-pyruvic transaminase, GPT);
- aspartate aminotransferase (glutamic-oxaloacetic transaminase, GOT);
- phosphohexose isomerase;
- phosphoglucomutase;
- α-hydroxybutyrate dehydrogenase;
- malate dehydrogenase.

Most of these are major 'soluble' (sarcoplasmic) muscle enzymes. Their increase in serum in DMD probably reflects increased efflux through the muscle membrane, possibly augmented later in the disease process by release from fibres undergoing necrosis. Evidence supporting this idea has been critically assembled by Rowland (1980), who also provides an extensive bibliography. The evidence may be summarized as follows.

1. The isoenzyme pattern of certain enzymes in serum closely resembles that of muscle tissue.

2. Under certain experimental conditions, it has been shown that enzymes are released from viable muscle tissue *in vitro*.

3. In patients aldolase levels have been shown to be slightly higher in the venous return than in the corresponding arterial supply of the lower limb.

4. Almost all of the enzymes that are increased in the serum of patients are cytoplasmic, whereas enzymes that are bound in some way to intracellular structures are not ordinarily found in the serum.

5. When the activity of an enzyme is increased in the serum of patients with DMD, it is almost always decreased in affected muscle, thus indicating that the enzyme originated from muscle.

6. The decline in serum enzyme levels as the disease progresses correlates well with the diminishing muscle mass.

7. Finally, the idea is further supported by the fact that, at least in some cases, release is related to molecular size. The molecular weights of CK (81 000 daltons or 81 kDa) and aldolase (150 kDa) are considerably less than in adenosine monophosphate (AMP) deaminase (320 kDa) and phosphofructokinase (400 kDa), which are also major muscle enzymes but which are virtually absent in serum of patients with DMD. However, some proteins with small molecular weights either do not appear at all in the serum of patients (adenylate kinase, 21 kDa), or only in relatively small amounts (myoglobin, 17 kDa).

The situation is therefore not simple and cannot be explained purely in terms of leakage from affected muscle. The serum level of an enzyme will be affected by its clearance rate, and its efflux from muscle will depend on its relative concentration in this tissue, its binding to intracellular structures, and possibly some form of selective force at the level of the muscle membrane but about which little is yet known.

From a practical point of view it is not possible to distinguish DMD and BMD on the basis of serum levels of various enzymes.

Muscle pathology

A great deal has been written about the pathology of muscle in various neuromuscular disorders. Several extensive monographs have been published that deal in detail with the various changes observed in the course of these diseases (Dubowitz 1985; Kakulas and Adams 1985; Karpati 2002). Here only a brief description will be given of those changes in muscular dystrophy that are helpful in establishing the diagnosis.

Biopsy technique

While in the past a lot of emphasis was put on the need to choose a moderately affected muscle, nowadays the availability of a direct protein test (the expression of dystrophin) allows a confident diagnosis to be made of DMD or makes it possible to differentiate it from other forms of dystrophy even in muscles that are pathologically only minimally affected. The choice of the muscle biopsy is therefore only determined by which muscle is safe and easy to access—this is usually the quadriceps.

In the past the method of open excision under general anaesthesia was the method of choice. This was despite the recognized anaesthetic risks in patients who often have compromised respiratory and cardiac function. Although Duchenne himself had advocated the use of a biopsy needle 100 years ago, for a long time this did not meet with favour, largely because of the fear that, being a 'blind' procedure, there might be the danger of damaging nerves or blood vessels. In fact, however, this has not proved the case and most now favour the use of a biopsy needle (Fig. 4.2) introduced with local anaesthesia under sterile conditions. The procedure can be performed safely even in young non-collaborative children. At the Hammersmith Hospital we have used with good success over the last 15 years oral sedation using choral hydrate or buccal or intranasal midazolam. This has the advantage of avoiding a general anaesthetic for children at risk of developing rhabdomyolysis and hyperkalaemia.

Excellent results are obtained with muscle frozen in liquid nitrogen-cooled isopentane and studies made on cryostat sections. The latter procedure is associated with fewer artefacts and has the advantage that histochemical and immunohistochemical studies can be carried out on the material. Transverse sections are more informative than longitudinal sections as they allow a better assessment of the variability in fibre size, internal nucleation, fibrosis, and degeneration and regeneration. Paraffin embedding of fixed material is no longer necessary, and this is an advantage because of the smaller quantity of muscle that can be obtained with a needle compared to that obtained with an open biopsy.

In a well established case of DMD, the changes observed in, say, the quadriceps or gastrocnemius muscles include increased variation in fibre size, fibre necrosis with phagocytosis, and, eventually, replacement by fat and connective tissue (Fig. 4.3). It is worthwhile considering some of these changes in a little more detail and tracing their development during the course of the disease.

Preclinical stage

Before there are any obvious clinical manifestations of the disease, there are already significant abnormalities in muscle pathology. Very early on the only significant abnormalities may be an increased variation in fibre size, and an increase in the number of prominent rounded fibres staining more densely

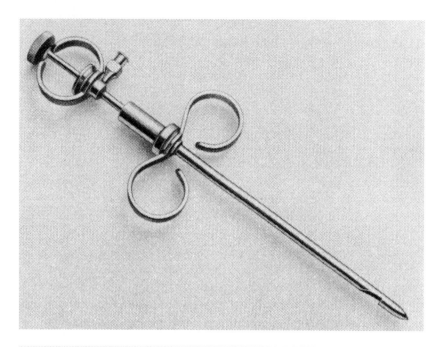

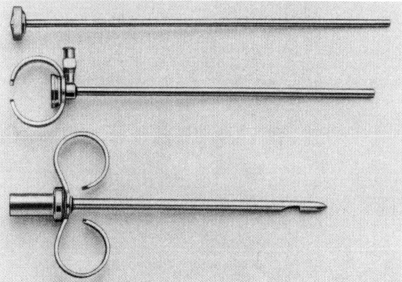

Fig. 4.2 The UCH skeletal muscle biopsy needle. (Above) The assembled instrument. (Below) The constituent parts which include the cutting cannula with a side arm for applying suction and the outer needle. (Instruments supplied by NI Medical, Redditch, Worcestshire, England.)

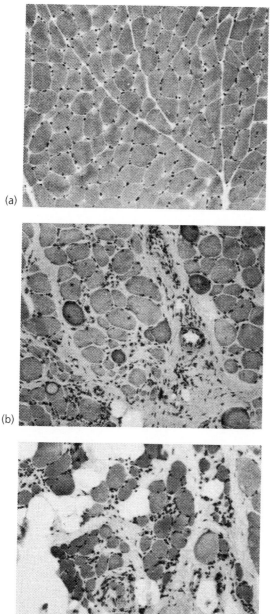

(a)

(b)

(c) 100µm

Fig. 4.3 Transverse cryostat sections of gastrocnemius muscle from: (a) a healthy boy; (b) an early case of DMD; (c) an advanced case of DMD. (Haematoxylin and eosin.)

with eosin—here referred to as eosinophilic fibres. In normal muscle these fibres are absent or very infrequent and, when present, they typically occur at the periphery of sections, indicating that they are artefactual.

On the other hand, in DMD, they are seen throughout sections and in some cases can be particularly frequent (Fig. 4.4). These same fibres contain increased intracellular calcium as revealed by histochemical staining with alizarin red S, or a fluorescent method with pentahydroxyflavone (Morin) (Fig. 4.5).

Increased intracellular calcium in skeletal muscle in DMD has been demonstrated not only histochemically but also by X-ray microanalysis and by chemical methods. The relevance of increased intracellular calcium in the pathogenesis of DMD will be discussed in Chapter 10 (p. 165 et seq.).

The proportion of calcium-positive fibres in DMD is very variable and the highest proportion has been found in a preclinical case (Table 4.1). A significant increase in calcium-positive fibres also occurs in BMD, but to a much lesser degree in other muscular dystrophies. The intracellular accumulation of calcium appears to be the prelude to the breakdown and death (necrosis) of the muscle fibre.

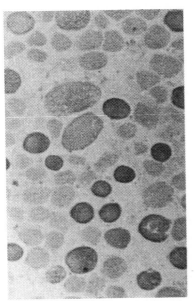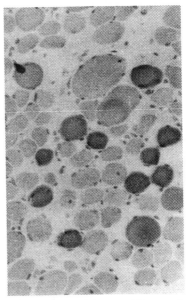

Fig. 4.4 Serial sections of gastrocnemius muscle in a preclinical (2-year-old) case of DMD stained with (left) haematoxylin and eosin and (right) alizarin red S. Note the numerous eosinophilic/calcium-positive fibres, but no evidence of muscle fibre necrosis.

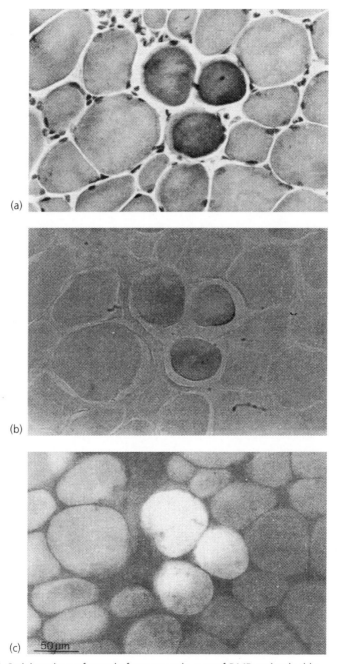

Fig. 4.5 Serial sections of muscle from an early case of DMD stained with:
(a) haematoxylin and eosin; (b) alizarin red S; (c) fluorescent Morin. (From Emery
and Burt (1980) with permission.)

Table 4.1 Proportion (%) of eosinophilic and calcium-positive fibres in crysotat sections of gastrocnemius muscle biopsy samples from boys with no neuromuscular disorder and boys with DMD (personal observation by one of the authors)

	Age (years)	Proportion (%) in cryostat sections of	
		Eosinophilic fibres	Calcium-positive fibres
Controls (N = 7)	5–12	<0.2	<0.1
DMD patients			
B103	10	6.0	5.8
B110	9	1.4	1.8
B115	7	3.0	2.9
B111	6	2.7	4.4
B106	5	4.1	6.5
B117*	3	3.7	53
B159*	2	15.3	18.3

* Preclinical cases.

At this early stage in the disease process, regenerating fibres are also commonly found. They are recognized by their smaller size in cross-section, basophilic cytoplasm, high concentration of ribonucleic acid (RNA), and large pale vesicular nuclei with prominent nucleoli. Other early changes are represented by focal areas of degeneration, with clusters of fibres undergoing degeneration/regeneration, at times affecting entire fascicles, and an increase in rounded fibres that are often hypercontracted. However, the process of regeneration becomes less frequent as the disease progresses and fibres undergoing necrosis become more obvious. For reasons that are not yet clear, muscle fibres of smaller diameter seem more resistant to necrosis.

Later stages

The changes that take place as a muscle fibre undergoes necrosis are complex. As the intracellular structures are destroyed the fibre is invaded by phagocytic cells. Often one can observe localized necrosis and degeneration of fibres segmentally invaded by phagocytic cells. Muscle fibres in various stages of degeneration and regeneration are illustrated in Fig. 4.6.

As the necrotic fibres are phagocytosed, they are replaced by fat and connective tissue so that eventually only small islands of muscle tissue remain. There is a significant pathological overlap between DMD and BMD, and a confident pathological diagnosis must rely on studies of dystrophin expression and not on simple morphological grounds.

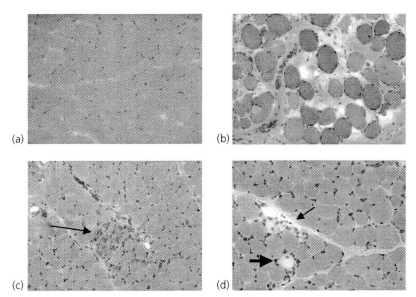

Fig. 4.6 (a) Normal muscle. (b) Duchenne muscle with hypercontracted fibres, abundant connective tissue, fat, and internal nuclei. (c) Duchenne muscle with cluster of basophilic regenerating fibres (arrow) and only mild fibrosis. (d) Duchenne muscle showing a small cluster of necrotic fibres (small arrows) and an isolated one (big arrow). See colour plate section in the centre of this book.

The histological changes in muscular dystrophy are very different from those in spinal muscular atrophy. In the latter group of disorders, all those muscle fibres associated with the defective neuron gradually atrophy. This produces the classical picture of group atrophy and is pathognomonic of spinal muscular atrophy (Fig. 4.7). The atrophy may be so profound as to present the appearance of 'nuclear clumps'. In spinal muscular atrophy, affected fibres undergo atrophy and tend to be grouped together. In contrast, in muscular dystrophy, affected fibres undergo structural changes and these occur in individual fibres at random. However, especially in the more chronic forms of neurogenic atrophy, muscle fibres adjacent to groups of atrophic fibres may undergo changes similar to those seen in muscular dystrophy: variation in fibre size, central nuclei, and even occasionally fibre necrosis and phagocytosis. It is possible that such changes result from faulty attempts at reinnervation: the metabolism of these abnormally innervated fibres is disturbed in some way that then results in the structural changes that might resemble a muscular dystrophy. Usually, however, significant fibrosis is not observed in neurogenic disorders. On the other hand, it is not uncommon to

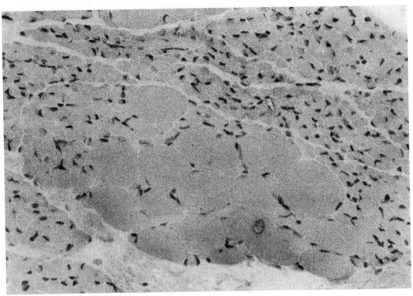

Fig. 4.7 Muscle fibre atrophy in spinal muscular atrophy (Werdnig–Hoffmann disease). Note large groups of atrophic fibres (Haematoxylin and eosin).

observe 'pseudoneurogenic' changes in the muscle biopsy of some of the chronic forms of muscular dystrophy. While this does not occur in DMD, it can be occasionally found in BMD and, more frequently, in facioscapulo-humeral and in Emery–Dreifuss muscular dystrophies. Various investigators have pointed out the problems that can be encountered in interpretation of the pathology. For example,

> . . . small, angular fibers can derive from fiber splitting, which can be the result of either a chronic myopathy, denervation, or tenotomy. Small groups of atrophic fibers can result from splitting or regeneration after necrosis. The changes described as characteristic of myopathy have been reported in biopsies from muscles affected by chronic denervation. (Bradley and Fulthorpe 1978)

In polymyositis there can also be muscle fibre necrosis and regeneration, but the distinctive pathological features in this disorder are the lack of hyper-trophic fibres and infiltration of muscle tissue by inflammatory cells (mainly lymphocytes and plasma cells). The latter is usually focal, around blood vessels and within muscle fibres. However, the distinction between groups of phago-cytic cells as seen in DMD and perivascular infiltrates of lymphocytes and plasma cells in polymyositis is not always clear. Furthermore, in childhood polymyositis/dermatomyositis, muscle histology may show only minimal changes or practically no significant changes at all. For this reason some advocate open biopsy in suspected polymyositis to ensure that as much tissue as possible can be examined.

More recently, the finding that human leukocyte antigen (HLA) class I is significantly upregulated at the sarcolemma in inflammatory myopathies but not in mature muscle fibres in DMD or other muscular dystrophies, has provided an additional and useful tool in the differential diagnosis. In particular upregulation of HLA class I at the sarcolemma may be the only change observed in inflammatory myopathies, even in the absence of other histological changes.

Muscle histochemistry

On the basis of physiological experiments in animals, and biochemical and histochemical studies on muscle tissue, it is possible to classify human skeletal muscle fibres into three distinct types, designated as 1, 2A, and 2B. Some of the differences between these fibre types are summarized in Table 4.2.

Animal experiments have shown that muscle fibres innervated by a single motor neuron possess similar physiological properties and identical histochemical characteristics. Thus, there would appear to be at least three types of motor neurons. Figure 4.8 shows the effects of denervation as it occurs in spinal muscular atrophy. If this is rapidly progressive there may be little time for reinnervation. However, if reinnervation occurs, from nerve fibres from another neuron, this will lead eventually to groups of atrophic fibres being of the same histochemical type.

The appearance of fibre type atrophy in a case of Werdnig–Hoffmann disease is shown in Fig. 4.9, in which type 2 fibres are predominantly affected. However, both fibre types can atrophy after denervation though most larger fibres tend to

Table 4.2 Some characteristics of various muscle fibre types in human skeletal muscle

	Type 1	Type 2A	Type 2B
Speed of contraction	Slow	Intermediate	Fast
Appearance (myoglobin content)	Dark	Dark	Pale
Size	Small	Intermediate	Large
Enzyme activities			
ATPase pH 9.4	+	+++	+++
ATPase pH 4.3	+++	+	+
Oxidative*	+++	++	+
Phosphorylase	+	++	+++

* NADH-tetrazolium reductase, succinic dehydrogenase.

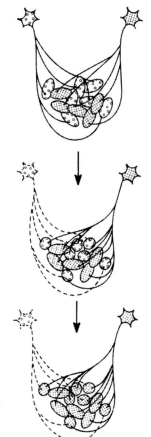

Fig. 4.8 Diagrammatic representation of the possible effects of denervation followed by reinnervation. For simplicity only two types of fibres are illustrated.

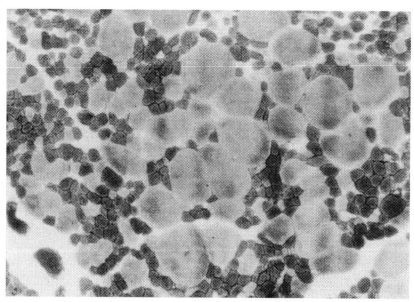

Fig. 4.9 Fibre-type atrophy in a case of Werdnig–Hoffmann disease (ATPase pH 9.4).

be of type 1. In muscular dystrophy and polymyositis no particular fibre type is predominantly affected and there is no grouping of fibre types.

The reason why certain groups of muscles are especially affected early in the course of muscular dystrophy is not at all clear. This presumably reflects some difference in their biochemical/physiological properties compared with muscles affected to a lesser degree and only in the later stages of the disease. Initial studies focused on the possibility that the selective involvement might be related to the different proportion of type 1 and type 2 fibres of different muscles. Johnson *et al.* (1973) in particular correlated the proportions of type 1 and type 2 fibres in normal skeletal muscles that in DMD are either severely affected or relatively unaffected. They found that there was a tendency for the proportion of type 2 fibres to be higher in muscles that are more severely affected, but there was no simple correlation between fibre-type composition of individual muscles and their being affected or spared in the disease. Using their extensive data, we calculated there would appear to be a slight excess of type 2 (or deficiency of type 1) fibres in those muscles affected early in the disease, but there is considerable variation, and the difference from those muscles affected later in the course of the disease is not statistically significant (Table 4.3). Whatever may be responsible for the differential involvement of muscles in DMD, it is not a simple matter of histochemical fibre type.

Muscle innervation

In addition to the indirect changes such as fibre-type grouping, a useful technique for studying denervated muscle is the intravital or supravital staining of motor nerve filaments and end-plates with methylene blue. The motor end-plate is a complex structure at the site where excitation is transmitted from the motor nerve to the muscle fibre (Fig. 4.10). In spinal muscular atrophy there is branching of subterminal intramuscular nerve fibres (Fig. 4.11) with collateral reinnervation, and degeneration of motor end-plates.

Branching of nerve fibres in this way is found in all forms of spinal muscular atrophy, but is very rarely seen in normal or dystrophic muscle.

Electron microscopy

Electron microscopy of muscle has provided details of the ultrastructural changes that take place in muscular dystrophy. These include distention of the sarcoplasmic reticulum, Z-band degeneration ('streaming'), and disruption and loss of myofilaments, followed later by complete disarray of the band structure (Fig. 4.12).

Table 4.3 Mean proportion (%) of type 1 and type 2 fibres in various normal human muscles (Johnson *et al.* 1973), which the present authors have divided into those muscles clinically affected early or late in the course of DMD

	Proportion (%) of fibres in normal human muscles	
	Type 1	Type 2
Affected early		
Sternomastoid	35.2	64.8
Pectoralis major (sternocostal)	43.1	56.9
Triceps		
Surface	32.5	67.5
Deep	32.7	67.3
Brachioradialis	39.8	60.2
Extensor digitorum	47.3	52.7
Extensor digitorum brevis	45.3	54.7
Latissimus dorsi	50.5	49.5
Iliopsoas	49.2	50.8
Gluteus maximus	52.4	47.6
Vastus medialis		
Surface	43.7	56.3
Deep	61.5	38.5
Rectus femoris		
Lateral head, surface	29.5	70.5
Lateral head, deep	42.0	58.0
Medial head	42.8	57.2
Tibialis anterior		
Surface	73.4	26.6
Deep	72.7	27.3
Mean	46.68	53.32
SD	—	12.74
Affected later		
Trapezius	53.7	46.3
Pectoralis major		
Clavicular	42.3	57.7
Biceps brachii		
Surface	42.3	57.7
Deep	50.5	49.5
Biceps femoris	66.9	33.1
Flexor digitorum brevis	44.5	55.5
Flexor digitorum profundis	47.3	52.7
Gastrocnemius		
Lateral head, surface	43.5	56.5
Lateral head, deep	50.3	49.7
Medial head	50.8	49.2
Soleus		
Surface	86.4	13.6
Deep	89.0	11.0
Mean	55.63	44.37
SD	—	16.42

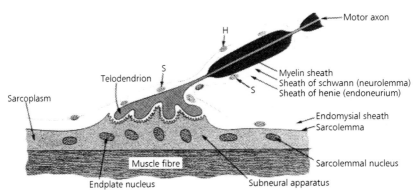

Fig. 4.10 The structure of the normal human end-plate. H, Nucleus of sheath of Henle; S, nucleus of sheath of Schwann.

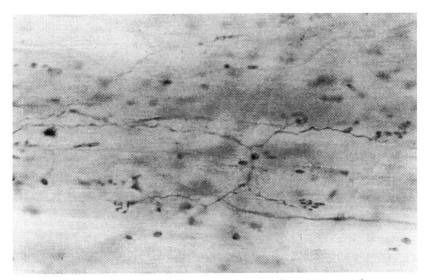

Fig. 4.11 Branching of subterminal intramuscular nerve fibres in a case of Wohlfart–Kugelberg–Welander spinal muscular atrophy (supravital staining with methylene blue).

These changes, however, are not specific to DMD but also occur in other forms of dystrophy. Various alterations in the sarcolemma have also been described early in the course of the disease, and include defects in the plasma membrane and reduplication of the basement membrane. These latter changes are common to conditions characterized by extensive degeneration and regeneration.

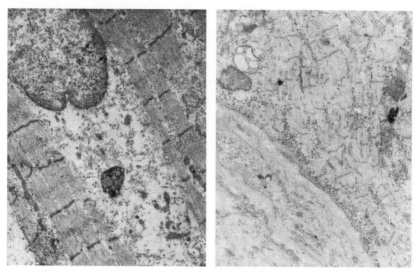

Fig. 4.12 Electron microscopy of skeletal muscle. (Left) Relatively early stage of DMD. The myofibrils have lost some myofilaments with widening of the intermyofibrillar space which contains a lysosome (phosphotungstic acid, ×14 000). (Right) Later stage showing disorganization of the band structure (2% uranyl acetate and lead citrate, ×7000). (Reproduced from Hughes (1974) with the kind permission of Dr. J. Trevor Hughes and Lloyd-Luke, publishers.)

DNA and dystrophin studies

The approach to the diagnosis of DMD and BMD has been revolutionized by the introduction of gene markers and dystrophin studies. In fact, some have argued that there is no place for any diagnostic investigations other than an SCK test (because of its simplicity, cheapness, and relative specificity) and DNA and dystrophin studies. However, as will become clear later, it is not always possible to predict with precision the phenotype resulting from mutations in the dystrophin gene by DNA analysis alone. The diagnostic approach that we recommend is therefore that of performing both a muscle biopsy for direct dystrophin studies as well as molecular genetic investigations to identify the primary genetic defect.

DNA studies on peripheral blood

As will be discussed in greater detail later, the gene locus for DMD and BMD has been located on the short arm of the X chromosome (at Xp2l). The mutation detection technique most commonly used in the first decade following the discovery of the dystrophin gene was the Southern blot, that is, the transfer of DNA after digestion with restriction enzymes, followed by hybridization with fragments of relevant genomic DNA (probes). With this technique it is possible to follow the inheritance of so-called restriction fragment length polymorphisms (RFLPs), which can be either close to the gene (extragenic) or actually within the gene (intragenic). In affected families, such linked RFLPs can therefore be used for tracking down the mutated chromosome X in a family by simply studying DNA obtained from peripheral blood (linkage analysis).

Unfortunately, because the gene is so large (approximately 3 megabases (mb)), not unexpectedly markers even within the gene may show recombination (cross-over) with a particular mutation and could therefore lead to misdiagnosis. It has been shown, for example, that polymorphic markers that lie at the two extremities of the dystrophin locus show a recombination frequency of 0.12 or 12 per cent. Using extragenic markers, the error rate can be even greater. This has therefore to be taken into account when using linked markers for diagnosis and the use of informative flanking markers is therefore recommended (see Chapter 11).

Another approach that does not require other affected members in the family in order to determine the so-called phase (see Chapter 11) of a DNA marker is to use a gene-specific (cDNA) probe. By using intragenic dystrophin probes, it is possible to determine if there is *a gene deletion or duplication*. Indeed, roughly 70 per cent of cases have a deletion or a duplication that can be detected on a Southern blot in this way.

An interesting finding is that deletions tend to be clustered around two 'hot-spot' regions (Fig. 4.13). Thus, the majority of deletions can be detected by examining only a subset of exons within the gene. In the late 1980s, Jeff Chamberlain and his colleagues (1988) and Alan Beggs *et al.* (1990) developed a method, referred to as the 'multiplex method', in which a number of regions (which are deletion-susceptible) are simultaneously analysed by amplifying these regions using the polymerase chain reaction (PCR). This important technique involves amplifying very small amounts of DNA such that eventually there is sufficient to visualize on a gel by fluorescence when stained with ethidium bromide. Particular regions of the DNA (in this case exonic regions most likely to be deleted) are amplified by PCR using primers that specifically flank these regions.

A diagrammatic example of the multiplex method is shown in Fig. 4.14. In family 1 the affected boy (B) has a deletion of exon *f* (as does a fetus (F) at risk in the same family); in family 2 the deletion is more extensive and involves exons *a–e* inclusive; in family 3 there is a deletion of exon *a* only. This is an extremely rapid method for screening for deletions and, by using two mixtures of primers, each of which amplifies nine exons, over 98 per cent of detectable deletions can be identified in this way. Since the introduction of

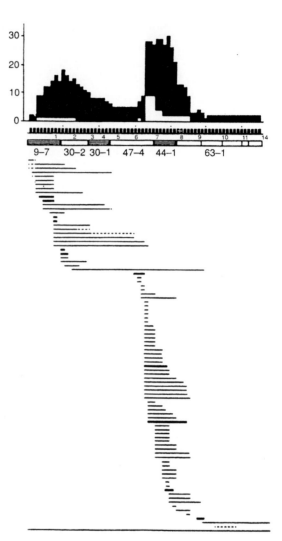

Fig. 4.13 Distribution and extent of gene deletions and duplications in DMD (solid) and BMD (open). (Reproduced by kind permission of Dr. E. Bakker and the publishers from Bakker (1989); copyright 1989, Wiley–Liss, a division of John Wiley and Sons.)

multiplex PCR, this technique has proved to be a rapid, reliable, and accurate method for detecting deletions. It requires only 1 day for analysis, with experience it is easy to perform, and, unlike Southern blot analysis, it does not require radioactive probes. The method, of course, cannot be used unless the patient being tested is related to an individual already known to carry a deletion detectable by the system.

If, as in family 4 in Fig. 4.14, there is no detectable deletion with this method, then resort has to be made to Southern blot analysis with full-length cDNA probes. The use of an automated and quantitative fluorescent PCR system has recently facilitated the detection of deletions, making it possible to assign the

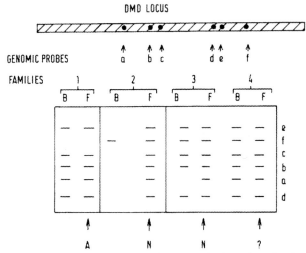

Fig. 4.14 Diagram of the results of the multiplex method used to simultaneously detect deletions in exons *a–f* in four families. B, Boy; F, fetus; A, affected; N, normal.

carrier status of females at risk. Moreover, more precise quantitation also allows the detection of duplications that were probably overlooked in the past using other techniques. Recent figures suggest that as many as 15 per cent of children carry a duplication of part of the gene.

But in roughly 20–30 per cent of cases, even with this detailed analysis, no deletion or duplication can be found. In these cases, the cause is a small mutation (point mutation or small deletion/ insertion; splice site mutation) or an intronic rearrangement or a promoter mutation. Various techniques have been used to look for those mutations that escape detection following the multiplex PCR approach. One technique (protein truncation test, or PTT) is based on an RNA strategy; the others are DNA-based techniques.

The PTT technique involves preparing total RNA from peripheral blood lymphocytes or, better, from muscle, which is then translated into protein in an artificial system. The large cDNA of the dystrophin gene is split into several small reactions and a resultant truncated protein fraction can be easily visualized on electrophoresis.

Regarding the genomic approaches proposed to detect mutation using genomic DNA, Mendell and his colleagues (2001) have used a very sensitive modification of the SSCP (single-strand conformation polymorphism) technique for identifying small mutations and deletions of the dystrophin gene from DNA obtained from blood. These authors studied 93 patients who had a clinical diagnosis of DMD confirmed on muscle biopsy, but in whom the standard multiplex PCR analysis had failed to recognize mutations. By this novel approach a mutation was identified in 73 of these 93 patients, therefore improving the ability to detect a mutation in DMD from ~65–70 to ~90 per cent of cases. The drawback of this technique is that each sample has to be run under different temperature conditions and, considering the large number of exons that comprise the dystrophin gene, even this technique, despite the possibility of its automation, is not very easily applicable on a large scale. By these various methods it is possible to detect deletions, duplications, and point mutations in the majority of cases and thus help in making diagnoses of both DMD and BMD. These genetic tests have their limitations, however, not only because mutations are not found in 100 per cent of cases, but also because the possibility of predicting the severity of the phenotype on the basis of the molecular findings is not absolute. The results of genetic testing need therefore to be complemented with the biochemical assay for dystrophin and, of course, the careful assessment of the patient.

Dystrophin studies on muscle biopsy material

The diagnosis of Xp2l myopathies, as DMD, BMD, and related muscle diseases are sometimes called, should also be established on the basis of studies of the gene product (dystrophin) in muscle biopsies. This is possible either by Western blot analysis or immunohistochemistry. The former involves separating proteins from a muscle extract on one-dimensional electrophoresis which is then 'blot probed' with various monoclonal antibodies to dystrophin. Using molecular weight markers, any difference from normal dystrophin (molecular weight 427 kDa) can be noted and the amount present semiquantified.

The results of such studies using various antibodies reveal a complete absence or only trace amounts of dystrophin in DMD. In BMD, on the other hand, dystrophin is present but in reduced amounts. Furthermore, in the latter disorder the dystrophin molecule is often of abnormal size, usually with a reduced molecular weight but occasionally with an increased molecular weight in the case of duplications.

Immunohistochemistry of cryostat sections of muscle provides another way of studying muscle dystrophin. In this method monoclonal antibodies to various parts of the dystrophin molecule (for example, the N-terminal, central rod, and C-terminal regions of the molecule) are raised in an appropriate animal and then labelled with a suitable marker (for example, peroxidase or fluorescent marker). This technique has revealed that, in normal muscle, dystrophin is located close to the sarcolemma, and ultrastructural studies indicate that it forms a lattice-like network adjacent to the membrane. The appearance on cryostat sections is shown in Fig. 4.15. This illustrates that, in

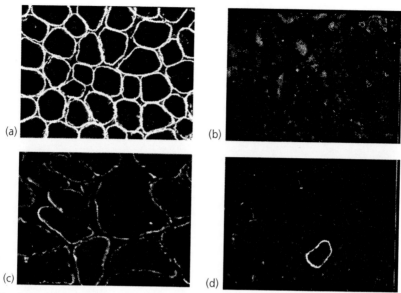

Fig. 4.15 (a) Dystrophin expression in control muscle. (b) Dystrophin in DMD, showing absent expression. (c) Dystrophin in BMD, showing reduced expression. (d) Dystrophin in DMD, showing a revertant fibre.

normal muscle, dystrophin is clearly localized at the periphery of muscle fibres. In DMD, however, the majority of fibres fail to show any staining at all. However, occasional fibres may show some labelling around the periphery. These positive fibres, so-called revertants, usually occur singularly but may be arranged in clusters, and are found in both familial and non-familial cases. Furthermore, using a panel of antibodies that span the entire dystrophin molecule, in patients with deletions the positive fibres only stain with antibodies raised to polypeptide sequences outside the deletion and not those within the deletion. These dystrophin-positive fibres are most probably the result of exon skipping that induces a restoration of the reading frame by creating larger in-frame deletions. Other mechanisms such as second-site in-frame mutation have also been proposed. In BMD most fibres do show some staining but this varies in intensity both between and within fibres. A list of antibodies commonly used in the diagnosis of DMD is indicated in Fig. 4.16.

A protein similar to dystrophin and referred to as dystrophin-like protein ('utrophin') has been identified and is synthesized by a gene on chromosome 6. This protein is normally concentrated in the region of neuromuscular junctions, myotendinous junctions, peripheral nerves, and vasculature of skeletal muscle but almost absent at the sarcolemma of mature muscle fibres, while it is highly expressed in the sarcolemma of fetal and regenerating fibres (Fig. 4.17).

ANTIBODIES TO DYSTROPHIN

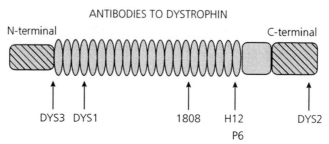

N-terminal   C-terminal

DYS3 DYS1   1808   H12   DYS2
                                         P6

Fig. 4.16 Scheme showing the various monoclonal (DYS 3, 1, 2) and polyclonal anti-dystrophin antibodies available.

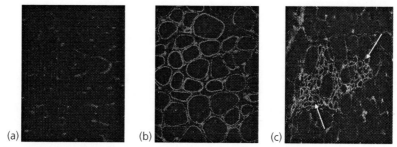

(a)   (b)   (c)

Fig. 4.17 Utrophin. (a) Normal muscle showing vascular tissue labelled but not sarcolemma. (b) DMD muscle with all fibres showing high sarcolemmal labelling. (c) BMD muscle showing groups of brightly labelled regenerating fibres (arrows) but also labelling on mature, larger fibres.

This protein is overexpressed at the sarcolemma in patients with DMD and BMD and its detection at the sarcolemma in non-regenerating muscle fibres is therefore a useful secondary indicator of a dystrophinopathy (Fig. 4.17).

In summarizing this section on dystrophin, Western blot analysis and immunohistochemistry on muscle tissue are important techniques for diagnosing a suspected case of Xp2l myopathy. In general, these two techniques complement each other.

From a practical point of view, immunohistochemistry is performed first. It can be performed on a few muscle sections, is rapid, and is reliable if appropriate controls are used. In particular, a marker protein to control for the preservation of the sarcolemma (such as, for example, β spectrin) should always be used (Fig. 4.18). Another important point is that multiple antibodies against dystrophin (not just one) have to be used. These have to be directed against different regions of dystrophin, and the most used are those against the *N*- and *C*-termini and the rod domain. The use of multiple antibodies increases the sensitivity of the changes observed but, even more importantly, it helps to

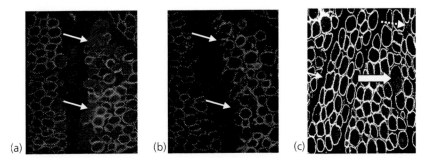

Fig. 4.18 Poor muscle preservation. (a) Dystrophin with loss of sarcolemmal labelling on some fibres (arrows). (b) Same fibres also show reduced β-spectrin due to damage (arrows). (c) DMD β-spectrin. Most fibres with normal sarcolemmal label, occasional necrotic fibre with very little spectrin (large arrow), and occasional regenerating fibre with reduced spectrin (dotted arrow).

differentiate DMD from BMD. In particular, it is important to realize that the presence of an in-frame deletion might give rise to a negative immunohisto-chemical result if the antibody used is raised against a deleted epitope. Only the immunohistochemical study with a panel of antibodies prevents misdiagnosis in these cases.

If dystrophin is absent or expressed only in trace amounts, there is no need to perform the Western blot analysis. However, if dystrophin is present but appears patchy and not strongly expressed at the periphery of muscle fibres, then a Westen blot may help to establish if the patient is affected by BMD.

If the size and abundance of dystrophin on Western blot and its distribution on immunohistochemistry are normal, then this excludes an Xp2l myopathy. A young patient with significant weakness and a muscle biopsy consistent with muscular dystrophy but normal dystrophin is very likely to have an autosomal recessive limb girdle muscular dystrophy of childhood.

The results of these investigations can also provide valuable information of prognostic value. Various studies have concluded that the probability of DMD exceeds 99 per cent if there is a complete absence of dystrophin, whereas the probability of BMD exceeds 95 per cent if dystrophin is present but of abnormal size (usually smaller) and/or reduced abundance. Patients with less than 20 per cent of normal levels of dystrophin tend to have an intermediate phenotype, becoming wheelchair-bound between the ages of 13 and 20 years. Minimal abnormalities of dystrophin expression have also been reported in cases of very mild, late-onset dystrophy as well as in exceptional healthy individuals with small in-frame deletions of the dystrophin gene. This widens the spectrum of expression of defects at Xp2l and will be discussed further in Chapter 9. An outline plan for investigating a suspected case of Xp2l myopathy is summarized in Fig. 4.19.

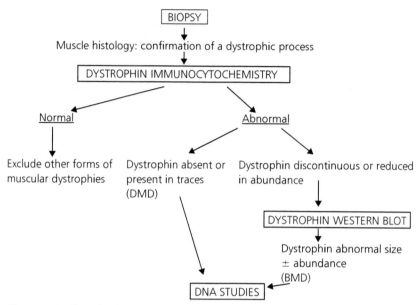

Fig. 4.19 Outline plan for investigating a suspected case of DMD.

Though muscle dystrophin studies can confirm the diagnosis, it is important to establish the precise molecular defect in a case if reliable prenatal diagnosis is to be offered in a future pregnancy of a female relative of the case.

Other investigations

The diagnosis of DMD can be established in all cases on the basis of the clinical findings, SCK level, and muscle biopsy for histology and dystrophin studies. In the past a lot of emphasis was placed on electromyography (EMG). However, a confident diagnosis of DMD can now be reached without an EMG. In a child who presents with proximal muscle weakness and markedly raised SCK levels and in whom the clinical picture does not support the possibility of a diagnosis of dermatomyositis, the most appropriate investigations are a muscle biopsy and genetic testing. An EMG is an unpleasant procedure, and does not help to distinguish DMD from other forms of muscular dystrophy.

Muscle ultrasound plays an important role in the investigations of childhood neuromuscular conditions. It has the advantages, compared to other techniques such as computerized tomography (CT scanning), of not being invasive and of being sufficiently sensitive to demonstrate and localize muscle loss by showing areas of changed density (Fig. 4.20). These imaging techniques are,

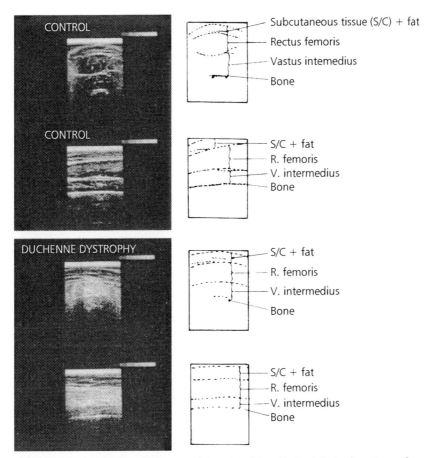

Fig. 4.20 Ultrasonogram of transverse (above) and longitudinal (below) sections of the thigh in a 7-year-old healthy boy and a boy with DMD of the same age. In the latter there is increased echogenicity throughout all the muscles. (Reproduced by kind permission of Dr Adnan Manzur and Professor Victor Dubowitz.)

however, unlikely to replace more conventional methods of establishing a diagnosis of muscular dystrophy.

Summary and conclusions

In the case of an otherwise healthy little boy who presents with evidence of proximal limb girdle muscle weakness and who has a grossly elevated SCK level (50–100 times normal), the diagnosis of DMD is almost certain. However, because of the importance of not missing an inflammatory myopathy that is treatable, and the need to exclude other disorders that can be inherited differently, a muscle biopsy is indicated in all cases. This is best carried out using a biopsy needle under local anaesthesia. The characteristic features of muscle histology are necrosis and phagocytosis of scattered individual muscle fibres in muscular dystrophy, muscle fibre group atrophy in spinal muscular atrophy, and infiltration with inflammatory cells (mainly lymphocytes and plasma cells) in polymyositis.

A significant feature of DMD is the presence of prominent, rounded fibres that stain densely with eosin, so-called eosinophilic fibres, which contain increased intracellular calcium. The immunostaining for dystrophin has to be performed using a panel of anti-dystrophin antibodies. If dystrophin is absent or present only in trace amount it is not necessary to perform further biochemical studies such as Western blot analysis.

Molecular genetic investigations will confirm the mutation in the majority of cases and this is essential for genetic counselling in the family and for prenatal diagnosis.

References and further reading

Bakker, E. (1989). Carrier detection and prenatal diagnosis of Duchenne/Becker muscular dystrophy by DNA-analysis. In *Genetics of neuromuscular disorders* (ed. C.S. Bartsocas), pp. 51–67. Alan R. Liss Inc., New York.

Beggs, A.H., Koenig, M., Boyce, F., and Kunkel, L.M. (1990). Detection of 98% of DMD/BMD gene deletions by polymerase chain reaction. *Human Genetics* **86**, 45–8.

Bradley, W.G. and Fulthorpe, J.J. (1978). Studies of sarcolemmal integrity in myopathic muscle. *Neurology* **28** (7), 670–7.

Bushby, K.M.D. and Anderson, L.V.B. (eds.) (2001). *Muscular dystrophy: methods and protocols*. Humana Press, Totowa, New Jersey.

Carpenter, S. and Karpati, G. (2001). *Pathology of skeletal muscle*, 2nd edn. Oxford University Press, New York.

Chamberlain, J.S., Gibbs, R.A., Ranier, J.E., Nguyen, P.N., and Caskey, C.T. (1988). Deletion screening of the Duchenne muscular dystrophy locus via multiplex DNA amplification. *Nucleic Acids Research* **16**, 11141–56.

Dreyfus, J.C., Schapira, G., and Démos, J. (1960). Étude de la créatine-kinase sérique chez les myopathies et leurs familles. *Revue Française Études Clinique et Biologie* **5**, 384–6.

Dubowitz, V. (1985). *Muscle biopsy: a practical approach*, 2nd edn. Baillière Tindall, Eastbourne.

Ebashi, S., Toyokura, Y., Momoi, H., and Sugita, H. (1959). High creatine phospokinase activity of sera of progressive muscular dystrophy. *Journal of Biochemistry* (*Tokyo*) **46**, 103–4.

Emery, A.E.H. and Burt, D. (1980). Intracellular calcium and pathogenesis and antenatal diagnosis of Duchenne muscular dystrophy. *British Medical Journal* **280**, 355–7.

Hughes, B.P. (1974). *Pathology of muscle*. Lloyd-Luke, London.

Johnson, M.A., Polgar, J., Weightman, D., and Appleton, D. (1973). Data on the distribution of fibre types in thirty-six human muscles—an autopsy study. *Journal of the Neurological Sciences* **18**, 111–29.

Kakulas, B.A. and Adams, R.D. (1985). *Diseases of muscle. Pathological foundations of clinical myology*, 4th edn. Harper and Row, Philadelphia.

Karpati, G. (ed.) (2002). In *Structural and molecular basis of skeletal muscle diseases*, pp. 6–19. ISN Neuropath Press, Basel.

Mendell, J.R., Buzin, C.H., Feng, J., Yan, J., Serrano, C., Sangani, D.S., Prior, T.W., and Sommer, S.S. (2001). Diagnosis of Duchenne dystrophy by enhanced detection of small mutations. *Neurology* **57**, 645–50.

Rowland, L.P. (1980). Biochemistry of muscle membranes in Duchenne muscular dystrophy. *Muscle and Nerve* **3** (1), 3–20.

Sibley, J.A. and Lehninger, A.L. (1949). Aldolase in the serum and tissues of tumor-bearing animals. *Journal of the National Cancer Institute* **9**, 303–9.

Chapter 5

Differential diagnosis

Disorders that could possibly be confused with Duchenne muscular dystrophy (DMD) include polymyositis, which must always be considered because it is treatable, other forms of muscular dystrophy that may present in early childhood, and, in particular, severe childhood autosomal recessive muscular dystrophy (SCARMD), a genetically heterogeneous group of disorders, various congenital dystrophies, and spinal muscular atrophy.

The congenital muscular dystrophies

This is very heterogeneous group of conditions. In all cases the disorder is evident at birth or within the first 6 months of life, with hypotonia and muscle weakness and frequent joint contractures. The muscle weakness is generalized, although some forms may affect the upper limbs more than the lower limbs and facial muscles are often affected. Tendon reflexes are usually reduced or absent and joint contractures may be present at birth or develop later in childhood. Intelligence is usually unimpaired in most of the variants that occur in the Western countries and all variants are inherited as autosomal recessive traits. A detailed description of each of the congenital muscular dystrophies goes beyond the scope of this book but further details can be found in the chapter on congenital muscular dystrophies in Mercuri and Muntoni (2001).

The forms that might be confused with DMD are essentially the primary deficiency of the laminin α2 chain of merosin, mapped to chromosome 6q (also known as MDC1A, for muscular dystrophy congenital 1A); a form with muscle hypertrophy linked to a yet unidentified gene on chromosome 1q and denominated MDC1B; and MDC1C, a recently identified form due to a defect in FKRP (Fukutin-related protein), a glycosyltransferase located on chromosome 19q. Interestingly, milder allelic variants exist of both MDC1A and MDC1C, and it is these later onset forms that may pose problems in the differential diagnosis of DMD.

The SCK levels are grossly elevated in all these variants, at levels comparable to those found in DMD.

The phenotype of the variant of MDC1A, characterized by total absence of the protein laminin α2, is more severe than DMD and affected children are never able to walk unsupported. A similarly severe phenotype is also characteristic of MDC1C, which is therefore relatively easily distinguishable from DMD. The confusion in the diagnosis is in cases of MDC1A with *partial* laminin α2 chain deficiency and a milder phenotype; or cases of MDC1B or milder cases of MDC1C. Helpful diagnostic hints for MDC1A (with either total or partial protein deficiency) are the presence of a mild demyelinating peripheral neuropathy and of a striking increase in the signal of the white matter on brain magnetic resonance imaging (MRI). The total absence of laminin α2 is diagnostic of the severe form of MDC1A. A partial protein deficiency is a feature of the milder end of the spectrum of MDC1A, but also of MDC1B and MDC1C. From a biochemical point of view, these forms also have a severe depletion of α-dystroglycan. Clinically, the brain and the peripheral nerve are never affected in MDC1B and MDC1C and the diagnosis can be confirmed on molecular genetic testing (Mercuri and Muntoni 2001).

Other X-linked muscular dystrophies

Over the years several other X-linked muscular dystrophies have been recognized, all relatively more benign than DMD. The commonest of these is Becker type muscular dystrophy (BMD), which occasionally presents in childhood when it can then be confused with DMD.

Becker type muscular dystrophy

This disease was first clearly delineated by Becker some 30 years ago (Chapter 2, this volume; Becker and Kiener 1955) but was recognized to be an allelic variant of DMD only after the identification of the dystrophin locus.

In contrast to DMD, BMD displays a wide range of clinical expression, ranging from individuals losing the ability to walk in the late teens, to individuals who may only experience mild proximal muscle weakness or cramps on exercise and never become significantly physically impaired during the course of their lives. Rare reports of individuals with isolated cardiomyopathy and 'typical' BMD deletions are on record, as well as a few families in which the only manifestation of a 'typical' BMD deletion was elevated SCK.

BMD is clearly less common than DMD, with a birth incidence of around 54×10^{-6} in the UK (Bushby *et al.* 1991; Emery 1991). In some populations, however (for example, in Sardinia and Malta, personal observation of one of the authors), the frequency of BMD appears to be higher, approaching that of DMD.

The distribution of muscle wasting and weakness is very similar to that in DMD and, as in DMD, the hip flexors and quadriceps muscles tend to be affected early in the lower limbs, while in the upper limbs the serrati, pectoralis, biceps, brachioradialis, and triceps muscles are usually affected first (Fig. 5.1).

Although weakness almost always begins in the lower limbs, eventually the upper limb musculature becomes affected. Calf enlargement is almost invariably present and contractures tend to be less severe than those in DMD. Cardiac involvement is a common manifestation, usually not present in the first 15 years of life, but eventually affecting some 60–65 per cent of patients. A small proportion of cases have some impairment of intellect. The SCK level is substantially raised, especially in the early stages, and gradually falls as the disease progresses. In the preclinical stage of BMD, when the only abnormality is calf enlargement and there is no apparent muscle weakness, the SCK level is grossly elevated to levels comparable to those found in boys with DMD of the same age but who are clinically affected.

The very high SCK levels early in the course of BMD and overlap in age in onset with DMD can present a diagnostic dilemma in isolated cases. Points of clinical value in distinguishing between the two disorders have been mentioned in Chapter 3 and essentially can be summarized as follows.

◆ Children with DMD are never able to run properly, hop on one leg, lift their head off the bed, or get up from a sitting position on the floor if asked to keep their arms folded.

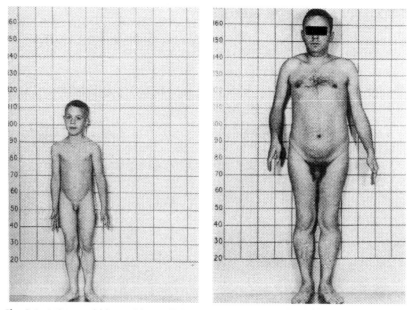

Fig. 5.1 A 6-year-old boy with preclinical BMD (note the enlarged calves) and his affected 26-year-old uncle.

+ Conversely, children affected with BMD are typically able to run, hop, can lift the head off the bed, and get up from the floor without Gowers' manoeuvre, at least in the early phases of the disease.

Later, the two disorders differ in the age of becoming confined to a wheelchair—in DMD this *usually* occurs by age 12, but in BMD after age 16. Many with BMD only become chairbound in late adult life and the reported mean age of loss of independent ambulation is 37 years (Bushby and Gardner-Medwin 1993).

Apparent DMD and BMD in the same family

The occurrence of patients with classical DMD and others with BMD within the same family is very rare. In at least one instance, a *de novo* independent additional mutation in the dystrophin gene has been reported in a child with DMD in a BMD family, providing the molecular basis for the discrepant phenotype. Another more common mechanism occurs in siblings with BMD with out-of-frame deletions where a discordant phenotype is the different occurrence of revertants generated by exon skipping (see Chapter 13 for a more detailed explanation on exon skipping). Exon skipping can induce a larger in-frame functional deletion, partially restoring dystrophin function (page 243, Chapter 13).

The diagnostic approach to differentiating DMD from BMD on clinical and biochemical grounds was discussed in Chapter 3.

X-linked muscular dystrophy with early contractures and cardiomyopathy (Emery–Dreifuss type)

In 1961, Dreifuss and Hogan described a large family in Virginia in the United States with an X-linked form of muscular dystrophy, which they considered at the time to be a benign type of DMD. However, on reinvestigating the family a few years later, this seemed to one of us to be a very different disease from either DMD or BMD, and a report setting out the differences was published in 1966 (Emery and Dreifuss 1966). The onset is in early childhood and is marked by progressive muscle wasting and weakness that, in the beginning, affects the lower limbs more than the upper limbs. The progression is relatively slow and most affected individuals survive into middle age with varying degrees of incapacity. There does not appear to be any intellectual impairment. The SCK level is usually slightly raised but even in the early stages never approaches the grossly elevated levels found in DMD. The distinctive features of this disorder are as follows (Emery 1989).

+ Early contractures of the elbows and Achilles tendons and later the posterior cervical muscles.

- Muscle weakness is more proximal (scapulohumeral) in the upper limbs and distal (anterior tibial and peroneal muscles) in the lower limbs, at least in the beginning.

- There is no calf pseudohypertrophy.

- Myocardial involvement with cardiac conduction defects is a frequent and important feature (Fig. 5.2). Provided the diagnosis is made sufficiently early, the insertion of a cardiac pacemaker can be life-saving.

The gene responsible for X-linked Emery–Dreifuss muscular dystrophy is the *STA* gene located in Xq28 and encoding for emerin, a nuclear envelope

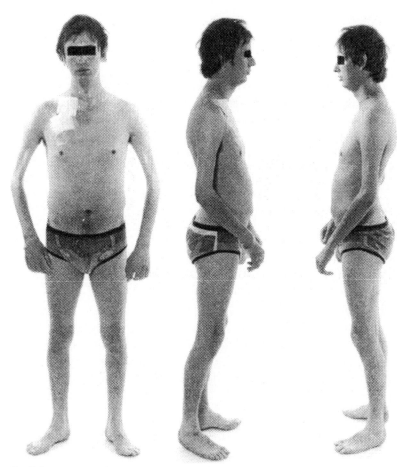

Fig. 5.2 A 17-year-old boy with X-linked muscular dystrophy with early contractures and cardiomyopathy. Note the flexion contractures of the elbows and wasting of the lower legs. A cardiac pacemaker has been inserted.

protein. The diagnosis of X-linked Emery–Dreifuss muscular dystrophy is based on the expression of emerin using immunocytochemistry in muscle or skin samples: in affected males typically there is no expression. The diagnosis should be confirmed by appropriate molecular genetic studies. Recently, the gene for an autosomal dominant phenocopy of the X-linked Emery–Dreifuss muscular dystrophy variant has been localized to chromosome 1q where the *LMNA* gene encodes another nuclear envelope protein lamin A/C. Mutations are usually dominant missense mutations, and the expression of the normal allele makes interpretation of the immunohistochemistry or Westen blot difficult. The diagnosis is therefore dependent on the identification of mutations in the *LMNA* gene. A rare severe autosomal recessive form due to mutations of the *LMNA* gene also exists. Mutations in this gene unexpectedly also result in isolated dilated cardiomyopathy with conduction system disease, or in partial lipodystrophy, or in autosomal recessive axonal neuropathy.

Autosomal recessive limb girdle muscular dystrophy of childhood

Several autosomal recessive limb girdle muscular dystrophies (LGMD) are clinically almost indistinguishable from DMD. They are mostly due to mutations in the sarcoglycan genes (α, β, γ, and δ, responsible for LGMD2D, LGMD2E, LGMD2C, and LGMD2F, respectively). These genes encode for four sarcolemmal proteins that are part of the dystrophin complex. It is therefore not entirely surprising that the phenotype of children with these disorders, also referred to as severe childhood autosomal recessive muscular dystrophy (SCARMD), is so similar to that of children with DMD.

There are, however, subtle clinical differences that can help to distinguish DMD from SCARMD on clinical grounds. Early motor milestones are typically delayed in DMD, while they are normal in children with SCARMD. While in DMD children are never able to run or jump, these functional abilities are usually preserved at the beginning in most patients with SCARMD. Intelligence is always normal in SCARMD, and height and head circumference are within the normal ranges. SCK levels are similar to those found in DMD.

The distribution of weakness is very similar but there are some differences. In SCARMD there is typically more significant scapular winging and weakness compared to DMD and more substantial weakness of the hip and trunk extensors, with an increased lordotic posture compared to that generally observed in children with DMD. Peroneal and tibialis anterior muscles are also more affected compared to those of children with DMD, and it is not unusual to observe foot drop in the ambulant phases of children with SCARMD. Quadriceps muscle is more affected than hamstrings in DMD, but the reverse is generally found in SCARMD.

Cardiac function is usually better preserved in SCARMD than in DMD, with the possible exception of LGMD2F, in which early and severe cardiomyopathy has been reported. This is of interest also considering that the δ-sarcoglycan gene is responsible for LGMD2F but also for the cardio-myopathic hamster, an animal model of dilated cardiomyopathy. Respiratory function is also better preserved in SCARMD compared to DMD. The main similarities and differences between DMD and SCARMD are summarized in Table 5.1.

The diagnosis ultimately depends on immunocytochemical and Western blot analysis of the sarcoglycan proteins, followed by molecular genetic testing of the relevant genes. It is important to be aware that dystrophin expression on immunocytochemistry can be secondarily depressed in patients with mutations in the β and δ sarcoglycan genes, probably because the lack of these two proteins causes a more significant destabilization of the complex.

Another form of autosomal recessive muscular dystrophy with clinical features very similar to those of DMD is LGMD2I, due to mutations in the fukutin-related protein gene. Affected patients may present in childhood with proximal weakness, calf hypertrophy, and marked elevation of SCK. Cardiac involvement in the form of dilated cardiomyopathy is also frequently observed in LGMD2I, making the clinical differential diagnosis between this form and both DMD and BMD more difficult.

A full discussion of the autosomal recessive limb girdle muscular dystrophies is found in Bushby *et al.* (2001).

Table 5.1 Main clinical features of Duchenne muscular dystrophy (DMD) and severe childhood autosomal recessive muscular dystrophy (SCARMD)

Clinical features	DMD	SCARMD
Calf hypertrophy	Common	Common
Weak foot dorsiflexion	Rare	Common
Lumbar lordosis	Moderate	Severe
Scapular winging	Mild	Moderate to severe
Intellect	Normal to mild mental retardation	Normal
SCK levels	>10 times normal	>10 times normal
Respiratory failure	Late teens	Late twenties

The manifesting carrier of DMD

Female relatives of boys with X-linked DMD may occasionally manifest certain features of the disease. Gowers, in 1879, reported an affected girl in a clearly X-linked pedigree (Case 8), the sister of an affected boy (Case 15), and an isolated case (Case 30). Since then there have been many similar reports, manifestations of the disease ranging from calf enlargement, through varying degrees of muscle weakness, to occasionally severe incapacity (Figs 5.3 and 5.4).

It has been estimated that between 5 and 10 per cent of carriers have some degree of weakness. But this may be slight and only elicited on careful clinical examination. Calf enlargement has often been emphasized but is, in fact, an unreliable sign. Actual measurements of calf size may reveal no significant difference between controls and definite carriers. Onset of weakness varies considerably and may develop in childhood or may not become evident until adult life, and the weakness may be progressive or remain static. In many ways the distribution of weakness resembles that seen in adult LGMD, but differs in that pseudohypertrophy is usually present, the weakness is often asymmetric, electrocardiographic abnormalities similar to those seen in affected boys can

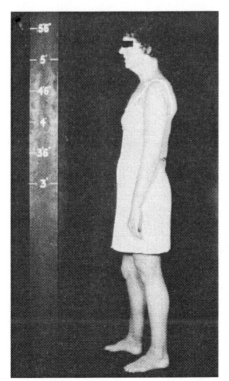

Fig. 5.3 A manifesting 36-year-old female carrier of DMD with lumbar lordosis, some enlargement of the calves, weakness of the anterior tibialis, quadriceps, and gluteal muscles, and, to a lesser extent, the shoulder girdle muscles. By age 47, weakness had progressed to such an extent that she became confined to a wheelchair.

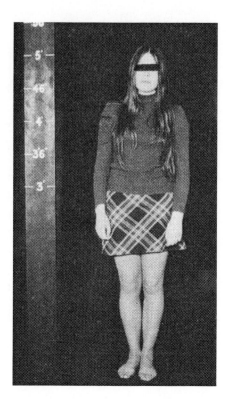

Fig. 5.4 A 19-year-old sister of a boy with DMD who has SCK levels in excess of 1500 IU and yet has no clinical manifestations of the disease.

occur, and the SCK level is invariably very high and occasionally may even approach levels found in affected boys. On the other hand, some female carriers may have very high SCK levels yet have no muscle weakness at all (Fig 5.4). Most importantly, the heart may also be affected and a proportion may develop a dilated cardiomyopathy even in the absence of any overt weakness (Grain *et al.* 2001).

It is important to distinguish a manifesting adult female carrier from a woman with autosomal recessive limb girdle muscular dystrophy (Table 5.2), both of which occur with very roughly the same frequency, because genetic counselling in these two situations will be quite different. The risks to the sons of a manifesting carrier of X-linked DMD will be 50 per cent, but the risks to the offspring of a woman affected with autosomal recessive limb girdle muscular dystrophy will be negligible. Manifesting carriers of BMD are exceptional.

Manifesting carriers of DMD have occasionally been described in the same family and this has also been observed in other X-linked disorders such as Fabry's disease (Fig. 5.5). DMD extending over seven generations has been described in a large Swiss family with 14 affected males and no fewer than four

Table 5.2 Differentiation between a manifesting carrier of DMD and a woman with limb girdle muscular dystrophy (LGMD)

Symptom or sign	DMD carrier	LGMD
Pseudohypertrophy	>80%	Rare*
Muscle weakness	Often asymmetric	Rarely asymmetric
ECG abnormalities (R-S in V1 increased)	5–10%	Usually normal
Dilated cardiomyopathy	5–8%	Usually normal*
SCK level elevated	>95% (often very high)	<50% (rarely high)
Muscle dystrophin	Mosaicism	Normal
Dystrophin DNA analysis	Abnormal	Normal

* With the exception of LGMD2I.

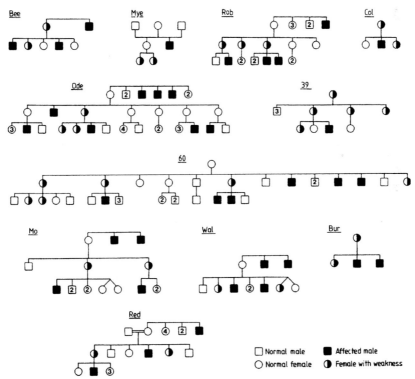

Fig. 5.5 Simplified pedigrees of families with DMD and several female relatives with weakness. Bee (Murphy and Thompson 1969); Mye, Rob, Col, and Ode (Moser and Emery 1974); 39 and 60 (Falcão-Conceição et al. 1983); Mo, Wal, and Bur (unpublished); Red (Reddy et al. 1984).

manifesting carriers. Since such manifestations are a consequence of random X-inactivation, their familial occurrence suggests that this process may be under genetic control. In fact, in the mouse there is an X-linked locus that controls X-inactivation (X-chromosome controlling element or Xce).

Such manifestations in heterozygous females can be explained in terms of random inactivation of the X chromosome. In those women with no clinical manifestations and a low SCK level, the active X chromosome in most cells is the one bearing the normal gene whereas, in those women with manifestations of the disease and a high SCK level, the active X chromosome in most cells is the one bearing the muscular dystrophy gene.

Manifesting carriers of DMD have a so-called mosaic expression of dystrophin in muscle. Such mosaicism, however, is rarely found in female carriers without symptoms. Mosaicism of dystrophin expression is believed to result from the formation of multinucleate muscle fibres from fusion of uninucleate myoblasts, in some of which the normal X chromosome is active (and therefore dystrophin-positive) while in others the abnormal X chromosome is active (and therefore dystrophin-negative). However, though some authors have hypothesized the existence of two distinct populations of muscle fibres in carriers, one normal and the other abnormal, a wide spectrum of abnormalities can be seen instead. These range from muscle fibres that appear to be normal through those that are clearly undergoing necrosis. The explanation lies in the way multinucleate muscle fibres originate and develop. If fetal myotomes were mosaics of nuclei in some of which the active X chromosome is the one bearing the normal gene and in others the active X chromosome is the one bearing the Duchenne gene, then fusion between mononucleate myoblasts derived from the myotomes would result in muscle fibres possessing different proportions of the two types of nuclei. The proportion in any one fibre would be determined to some extent by the proportion in the original myotome. The proportion of nuclei in any muscle fibre in which the active X-chromosome is the one bearing the Duchenne gene presumably determines the degree of abnormality in that fibre (Fig. 5.6).

This interpretation has been recently confirmed by detailed immunohistochemical studies on dystrophin expression. Abnormal dystrophin expression can be clearly identified in manifesting carriers, who often show a population of entirely dystrophin-negative fibres, of dystrophin-positive fibres, and a third, mixed population with variable levels of expression of dystrophin (see Chapter 11, p. 180 et seq.).

But, in non-manifesting carriers, variability in immunostaining is infrequent and negative fibres are rare, especially if the SCK level is normal. Interestingly, utrophin is also often upregulated in muscle fibres of carriers, despite the

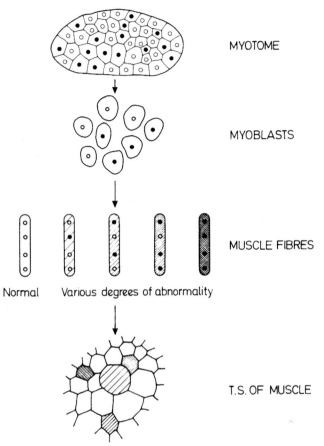

MYOTOME

MYOBLASTS

MUSCLE FIBRES

Normal   Various degrees of abnormality

T.S. OF MUSCLE

Fig. 5.6 Possible explanation for the muscle histological findings in carriers of DMD. (Open circles) Nuclei in which the active X chromosome bears the normal gene; (black circles) nuclei in which the active X chromosome bears the Duchenne gene. T.S., Transverse section.

apparent normal level of dystrophin, and therefore represents an additional marker that should be studied.

It is important to emphasize that secondary abnormalities of dystrophin immunostaining have been noticed in several cases of patients with sarco-glycanopathy and, in particular, in cases with mutations in the β and δ sarco-glycan genes. In a symptomatic female patient without a clear mosaic pattern of dystrophin expression, therefore, one of the recessive sarcoglycanopathies cannot be excluded. Further helpful hints come from the upregulation of utrophin, which is usual in cases of Xp21 muscular dystrophies but not in sarcol-glycanopathies (Fig. 5.7).

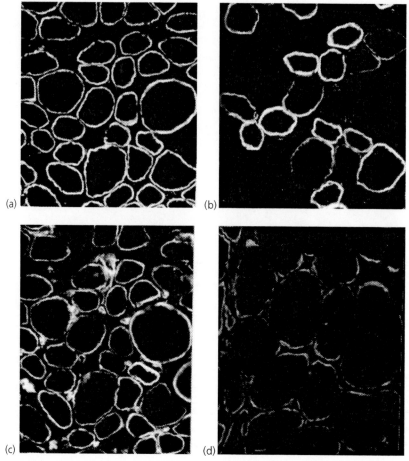

Fig. 5.7 (a)–(c) Duchenne carrier. (d) β-Sarcoglycanopathy. (a) Regular β spectrin expression indicating good sarcolemmal preservation. (b) Dystrophin-positive and -negative fibres in a DMD carrier. (c) Utrophin expression in all fibres in a DMD carrier. (d) Secondary reduction of dystrophin in a patient with β-sarcoglycanopathy.

Heterozygous identical twins

Over the years a number of female identical (monozygotic, MZ) twins have been described who are discordant for manifestations for various X-linked recessive disorders, most notably DMD, but also colour blindness, haemophilia B, G-6-P-D deficiency, and Hunter's disease. The simplest explanation is that, during the process of twinning, by chance the affected twin received a greater proportion of cells in which the active X chromosome was the one bearing the mutant gene. Certainly, there is experimental evidence that, in these cases, the clinical expression of the disease in the affected twin is the consequence of the inactivation of the normal X chromosome in most of her cells as compared with those of her unaffected twin sister. But why is the expression limited to only one twin of a pair and why is concordant expression in MZ heterozygous female twins extremely uncommon? This may be because the twinning event occurs after X-inactivation and, in these cases, in some way, non-random X-inactivation itself causes the twinning process. But discordance in female MZ twins has also been reported in certain autosomal disorders. The situation is therefore not clear. Lubinsky and Hall (1991) suggest that genomic imprinting, monozygous twinning, and X-inactivation may all be somehow related and '. . . their interactions may provide important clues to the nature of early developmental processes'.

The spinal muscular atrophies

The spinal muscular atrophies are defined as a group of inherited diseases in which there is degeneration of the anterior horn cells (lower motor neurons) of the spinal cord and often the bulbar motor nuclei, but with no evidence of pyramidal tract or peripheral nerve involvement. This group of diseases excludes motor neuron disease (progressive bulbar palsy, progressive muscular atrophy, and amyotrophic lateral sclerosis) and its variants, as well as the peripheral neuropathies. The spinal muscular atrophies (SMA) are a heterogeneous group of disorders and vary considerably in their clinical presentation and mode of inheritance. Distal and proximal variants are recognized, but the most common form is the chromosome 5-linked form of proximal spinal muscular atrophy, due to mutations in the *SMN* gene. This can be subdivided into several variants depending on disease severity. In type I (also known as Werdnig–Hoffmann disease) affected children present at birth or in the first 6 months and are never able to sit. In type II, children present before the eighteenth month of life and can sit but cannot walk. In type III (also known as Kugelberg–Welander disease), in which onset is usually after the eighteenth month of life, ambulation is possible. Some authors also recognize a fourth type with onset after the age of 30 years (SMA IV). These four subtypes are allelic, that is, due to mutations in the same gene, the *SMN* gene. Table 5.3 summarizes the main features of these common forms of SMA.

From a practical point of view, the only form that might possibly be confused with DMD is type III SMA (Fig. 5.8). The clinical presentation may closely resemble that of DMD: weakness first affects the pelvic girdle musculature and patients often present with a tendency to fall and a waddling gait. Later, the pectoral girdle, neck, trunk, and distal limb muscles also become

Table 5.3 Distinguishing features of the different forms of proximal spinal muscular atrophy (SMA)

Type	Age (usual)		Ability to sit without support	Muscle fasciculations	SCK
	Onset	Survival			
I (Infantile)	<6 months	<2 years	Never	+/−	Normal
II (Intermediate)	<18 months	Variable *	Yes	+/−	Usually normal
III (Juvenile)	>18 months	Adulthood	Yes	++	Often raised
IV (Adult)	>30 years	Normal	Yes	++	Often raised

* Survival into adolescence and adulthood increasingly possible.

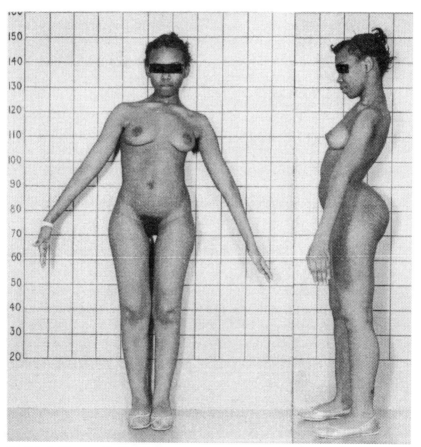

Fig. 5.8 A 17-year-old girl with type III spinal muscular atrophy (Wohlfart–Kugelberg–Welander disease). Note the marked lordosis and wasting of the left deltoid muscle. An older and two younger brothers were also affected.

affected. Interestingly, muscle weakness, at least in the early stages, is often asymmetric, which is unlike muscular dystrophy, pseudohypertrophy of the calf muscles is uncommon, and muscle fasciculations are often present and are a useful diagnostic sign. A fine tremor of the outstretched hands is common and minipolymyoclonus, intermittent and irregular movement that is sufficient to produce visible movement of the joints and head, may also be present. The progression of the disease is very variable, even within families, although the majority require a wheelchair in their twenties or thirties. The SCK level is very rarely grossly elevated, but it can be moderately elevated. In most cases electromyography confirms the neurogenic nature of the disorder. An useful sign is the presence of trembling of the electrocardiogram (ECG) baseline, due to fasciculation of intercostal muscles. The diagnosis of spinal muscular atrophy type III can now be rapidly and confidently established by DNA analysis, as more than 90 per cent of affected individuals have a mutation affecting the telomeric version of the *SMN* gene (also known as *SMN1* gene).

Summary and conclusions

Several disorders can mimic DMD. They include certain other forms of muscular dystrophy that may present in early childhood, various congenital muscular dystrophies, and a mild form of spinal muscular atrophy (SMA III). Among the muscular dystrophies, the congenital forms are unlikely to lead to confusion because, in general, they are evident at birth or in the neonatal period with severe hypotonia and generalized muscle weakness. However, milder allelic variants of some of these do overlap from a clinical point of view with both DMD and limb girdle muscular dystrophies. The best example is given by mutations in the *FKRP* gene, located on chromosome 19, responsible both for a form of congenital muscular dystrophy (MDC1C) and a form of limb girdle muscular dystrophy (LGMD2I) that presents with proximal muscle weakness, calf and thigh hypertrophy, grossly elevated SCK, and, frequently, a dilated cardiomyopathy. Among the other X-linked muscular dystrophies, the benign form associated with early contractures and conduction system disease (Emery–Dreifuss muscular dystrophy) is so distinctive clinically that this too is unlikely to cause confusion. But, because of the very high SCK levels early in the course of the disease, overlap in age at onset, and similar pattern of muscle involvement, BMD can present a diagnostic dilemma in the isolated case. However, an important point of distinction is that, in BMD, the abilities to lift the head off the bed, to run and hop, and to get up from the floor without the classical difficulties observed in DMD are preserved in the early phases of the disorder. Furthermore, muscle dystrophin is virtually absent in DMD, whereas in BMD dystrophin is present but abnormal.

A particularly difficult problem is posed by severe childhood autosomal recessive muscular dystrophy (SCARMD) when only a boy is affected in the family. One can suspect a severe autosomal recessive limb girdle muscular dystrophy in a child with normal early motor milestones and intelligence, significant scapular winging and weakness, and significant hip extensor and peroneal muscle weakness. The incidence of severe autosomal recessive limb girdle muscular dystrophy is, however, extremely low compared to DMD in most ethnic groups, and muscle immunohistochemical studies will confirm which protein is primarily involved, suggesting the final diagnosis that will eventually be confirmed by the appropriate molecular genetic investigations.

Finally, the only form of spinal muscular atrophy that might possibly be confused with DMD is the proximal juvenile form (type III, Kugelberg–Welander disease). Points that would suggest this disease rather than DMD would be some asymmetry of muscle involvement, absence of pseudohypertrophy, and evidence of muscle fasciculations. SCK levels are significantly (5–10 times normal) elevated in rare cases but more frequently normal. In most cases electromyography and muscle histology will confirm the neurogenic nature of the disorder. And again molecular genetic testing will confirm the diagnosis.

References and further reading

Becker, P.E. and Kiener, F. (1955). Eine neue X-chromosomale Muskeldystrophie. *Archiv für Psychiatric und Nervenkrankheiten* 193, 427–48.

Bushby, K.M. (2001). The limb-girdle muscular dystrophies. In *The muscular dystrophies* (ed. A.E.H. Emery), pp. 109–36. Oxford University Press, Oxford.

Bushby, K.M., Thambyayah, M., and Gardner-Medwin, D. (1991). Prevalence and incidence of Becker muscular dystrophy. *Lancet* 337 (8748), 1022–4.

Bushby, K.M. and Gardner-Medwin, D. (1993). The clinical, genetic and dystrophin characteristics of Becker muscular dystrophy. I. Natural history. *Journal of Neurology* 240 (2), 98–104.

Bushby, K.M., Gardner-Medwin, D., Nicholson, L.V., Johnson, M.A., Haggerty, I.D., Cleghorn, N.J., Harris, J.B., and Bhattacharya, S.S. (1993). The clinical, genetic and dystrophin characteristics of Becker muscular dystrophy. II. Correlation of phenotype with genetic and protein abnormalities. *Journal of Neurology* 240 (2), 105–12.

Dreifuss, F.E. and Hogan, G.R. (1961). Survival in X-chromosomal muscular dystrophy. *Neurology* 11, 734–7.

Emery, A.E.H. (1989). Emery Dreifuss syndrome. *Journal of Medical Genetics* 26, 637–41.

Emery, A. (1991). Population frequency of inherited neuromuscular diseases—a world survey. *Neuromuscular Disorders* 1, 19–29.

Emery, A.E.H. and Dreifuss, F.E. (1966). Unusual type of benign X-linked muscular dystrophy. *Journal of Neurology, Neurosurgery and Psychiatry* 29, 338–42.

Falcão-Conceição, D.N., Pereira, M.C.G., Gonçalves, M.M., and Baptista, M.L. (1983). Familial occurrence of heterozygous manifestations in X-linked muscular dystrophies. *Brazilian Journal of Genetics* **6**, 527–38.

Gowers, W.R. (1879). *Pseudo-hypertrophic muscular paralysis—a clinical lecture.* J. and A. Churchill, London.

Grain, L., Cortina-Borja, M., Forfar, C., Hilton-Jones, D., Hopkin, J., and Burch, M. (2001). Cardiac abnormalities and skeletal muscle weakness in carriers of Duchenne and Becker muscular dystrophies and controls. *Neuromuscular Disorders* **11**, 186–91.

Hilton-Jones, D. (2001). In *Disorders of voluntary muscle*, 7th edn (ed. G. Karpati, D. Hilton-Jones, and R.C. Griggs). Cambridge University Press, Cambridge.

Lubinsky, M.S. and Hall, J.G. (1991). Genomic imprinting, monozygous twinning, and X inactivation. *Lancet* **337** (8752), 1288.

Mercuri, E. and Muntoni, F. (2001). Congenital muscular dystrophies. In *The muscular dystrophies* (ed. A.E.H. Emery), pp. 10–38. Oxford University Press, Oxford.

Moser, H. and Emery, A.E.H. (1974). The manifesting carrier in Duchenne muscular dystrophy. *Clinical Genetics* **5**, 271–84.

Murphy, E.G. and Thompson, M.W. (1969). Manifestations of Duchenne muscular dystrophy in carriers. In *Progress in neurogenetics* (ed. A. Barbeau and J.R. Brunette), pp. 162–8. Excerpta Medica, Amsterdam.

Reddy, B.K., Anandavalli, T.E., and Reddi, O.S. (1984). X-linked Duchenne muscular dystrophy in an unusual family with manifesting carriers. *Human Genetics* **67**, 460–2.

Swash, M. and Schwartz, M.S. (1997). *Neuromuscular disorders*, 3rd edn. Springer Verlag, London.

Chapter 6

Involvement of tissues other than skeletal muscle

The muscular dystrophies have often been described as primary diseases of muscle. The term 'primary' in this context could have two interpretations—either that muscle is the most obviously affected tissue, which is certainly true, or that the fundamental molecular defect is expressed only in skeletal muscle, which is patently not true. In recent years it has been shown that significant abnormalities can be found in a variety of tissues quite apart from skeletal muscle. This is perhaps not unexpected since the abnormal gene is transcribed in a variety of cells of the body.

The variety of manifestations of a genetic disease can result from the pleiotropic effects of a single gene or, at the molecular level, either from the involvement of adjacent genes that control other phenotypic features or from different point mutations within the same gene.

Pleiotropy refers to the multiple effects that a gene mutation may have as a trail of consequences leading on from the basic defect. An excellent example of this is provided by sickle cell anaemia wherein the responsible gene mutation results in sickle cell haemoglobin, which is less soluble than normal haemoglobin and therefore tends to crystallize out resulting in deformation of the red cell, which becomes sickle-shaped. These abnormal cells are then destroyed (haemolysed) resulting in anaemia. But at the same time they also tend to clump together, thereby obstructing small arteries, resulting in ischaemia of tissues with a variety of consequences including attacks of abdominal pain, splenic infarction, limb pains, osteomyelitis, cerebrovascular accidents, haematuria, renal failure, 'pneumonic' episodes, and heart failure. While most of the features of DMD can be accounted for by the defect of dystrophin in the target tissue (that is, the absence of dystrophin in skeletal muscle is related to the development of the muscle damage; the absence of dystrophin in the cardiac muscle is related to the cardiomyopathy; the abnormal expression of dystrophin in brain is clearly involved in the mental retardation observed in affected children), some manifestations of disease are not so easily explained. For example, the development of muscle degeneration is not simply the result of dystrophin deficiency. The absence of dystrophin in facts triggers a *complex cascade of events* that includes muscle degeneration.

An association of different genetic disorders in the same individual can occur purely by chance, such as the reported occurrence in Duchenne muscular dystrophy (DMD) of haemophilia, trisomy-21, or facioscapulohumeral muscular dystrophy. However, very occasionally, such an association may result from the deletion of genetic material involving adjacent genes that are responsible for different diseases (contiguous gene syndrome or overlapping phenotypes). Several associations of DMD with disorders due to genes closely located on Xp21 have been described. These include a boy with DMD with chronic granulomatous disease and retinitis pigmentosa and another with DMD, glycerol kinase deficiency, and adrenal insufficiency. Often, cytogenetic studies reveal that these children have a small but visible interstitial deletion of the short arm of the X chromosome (Xp21) that involved the loss of genetic material from all three of the adjacent genes responsible for these different diseases (see Chapter 9, p. 142 et seq.). However, this sort of molecular abnormality is rare and very much the exception. A significant part of the variability observed in clinical practice among different children with DMD is due to differences in the site and extent of mutations within the dystrophin gene at Xp21.

Whatever the mechanism, it is important in patient management to appreciate that DMD is a multisystem disease and that a variety of tissues other than skeletal muscle can be affected. It is also important in genetic counselling to acquaint would-be parents with the possible consequences of the disease in an affected child so that they can better appreciate the full extent of the problem.

Smooth muscle

Circumstantial evidence that smooth muscle may be affected in DMD comes from the occasional occurrence of bladder paralysis, paralytic ileus, and gastric dilatation in affected boys. In addition, severe constipation is a frequent complication of the late phases of the disease. More direct evidence is provided by detailed autopsy studies that have shown that the smooth muscle of the gastrointestinal tract often shows variation in fibre size, atrophy and loss of muscle fibres, and areas of fibrosis. These changes are comparable in many ways to those seen in affected skeletal muscle and have occasionally been found in cases who did not have any relevant gastrointestinal symptoms in life. However, no lesions of the smooth muscle of the vascular system have so far been reported. From a functional point of view, however, children with DMD are known to suffer much more severe blood loss following major surgery, such as spinal surgery, compared to that experienced by other disease controls. In the absence of a clotting problem in these patients, it has been hypothesized (but not proved) that this abnormality is the result of the difficulty in arterial and arteriolar vasoconstriction of children with DMD.

Cardiac muscle

There is overwhelming evidence from clinical, pathological, and physiological studies that cardiac muscle is involved in DMD.

From an early age (already at presentation) there is very often a persistent sinus tachycardia and arrhythmias. Clinically apparent cardiomyopathy, however, usually first becomes evident with the loss of independent ambulation and increases in incidence with age thereafter. Mitral valve prolapse has been recorded in up to a quarter of affected boys, auscultatory evidence of which can be confirmed by echocardiography. While it is estimated that almost all DMD patients have signs of cardiac involvement in the late stages of their disease, progressive heart failure is rare (approximately 15 per cent of cases). Plasma atrial natriuretic peptide levels have been suggested as a means of evaluating cardiac function in the disease, as in other cardiomyopathies.

At autopsy, microscopic studies of cardiac muscle reveal features that resemble those seen in skeletal muscle with variation in fibre size, fragmentation of muscle fibres, replacement by connective tissue, and some fatty infiltration. Such changes have even been found in patients who did not necessarily have any symptoms of heart disease during life. Fibrosis appears to be a particularly important feature (Fig. 6.1). It begins in the outer myocardium involving the more posterobasal part of the outer free wall of the left ventricle. At first fibrosis appears in discrete small areas, but eventually becomes more diffuse and involves most of the outer half of the ventricular wall. The right ventricle and atria are rarely involved and this pattern of myocardial fibrosis does not seem to occur in any other disease except Becker muscular dystrophy (BMD) and X-linked dilated cardiomyopathy.

Early in the course of the disease, cardiac catheterization studies have shown few consistent abnormalities, but, in severely affected boys approaching cardiac failure, significantly elevated right atrial and right ventricular end-diastolic pressures have been recorded. Non-invasive techniques such as ballistocardiography, vectorcardiography, echocardiography, and, more recently, tissue Doppler studies have all documented variable degrees of cardiac involvement. With this latter technique, significant abnormalities can already be demonstrated in the early ambulant phases of the disease. Electrocardiography (ECG) has been used extensively over the years and therefore merits some special consideration. The first description of ECG abnormalities in muscular dystrophy dates back to 1929. Since then a variety of ECG changes have been observed and are

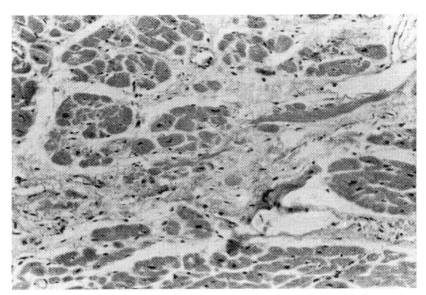

Fig. 6.1 Histological appearance of cardiac muscle from the left ventricle from a 21-year-old boy with DMD. Note the variation in fibre size and marked increase in connective tissue. (Haematoxylin and eosin.)

Table 6.1 ECG abnormalities arranged in decreasing order of frequency in DMD

Tall R waves in V_1
  R/S ratio $\uparrow$
  [R–S] $\uparrow$

Shortened P–R interval
Deep Q waves in V_{5-6}
Complex RSr[1], right bundle branch block
Altered T waves
Left axis deviation

listed in Table 6.1. Evidence of defective cardiac conduction has also been reported.

Numerous attempts have been made to determine if any particular ECG pattern is specific to DMD. Ishikawa and his colleagues in Japan (1982) have suggested that high-frequency 'notches' on the QRS complexes can be used for estimating the extent and severity of cardiac involvement in DMD. Shortening of the PQ interval has been found to be particularly valuable in this respect. There is also general agreement that the presence of tall R waves in V_1 is a

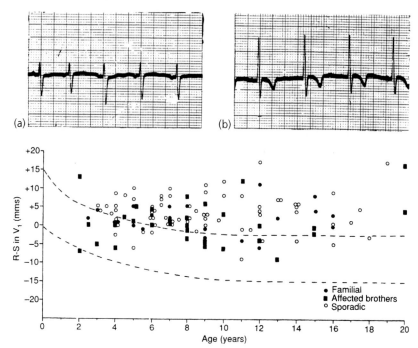

Fig. 6.2 Right praecordial lead (V_1) in: (a) a healthy boy and (b) a boy with DMD, both aged 10. Algebraic sum of R–S in V_1 for boys with DMD. Normal 90% confidence limits from Nadas (1963, p. 71). (Taken with permission from Emery (1972).)

particularly frequent and consistent abnormality in the disease. A useful measure of this is the algebraic sum of the R and S waves in this lead (that is, [R–S] in V_1), which is abnormal in over 80 per cent of affected boys (Fig. 6.2). It is particularly interesting that the same abnormality has also been found in up to 10 per cent of female carriers of the disease, while it is uncommon in other childhood forms of dystrophy.

The aetiology of the tall R waves in the right praecordial lead of the EGG is not clear. Various suggestions have been made including thoracic deformity, pulmonary hypertension, conduction defect due to myocardial dystrophy, and ventricular septal hypertrophy.

However, none of these suggestions is entirely satisfactory. It seems that this anterior shift of the QRS complex is most probably due to the diffuse interstitial fibrosis in the posterobasal part of the left ventricle (Fig. 6.3). Involvement of the adjacent papillary muscle would account for mitral valve prolapse that can occur in the disease. Evidence supporting this idea comes from necropsy findings, which have already been discussed, and also from echocardiography.

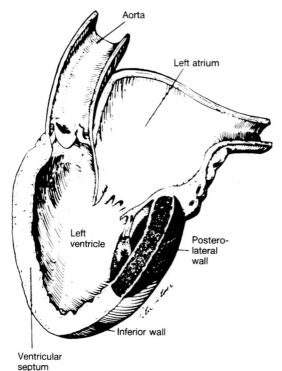

Fig. 6.3 Diagram of the left side of the heart illustrating the region of selective involvement in DMD patients. (Reproduced from Perloff *et al.* (1966) by kind permission of Dr J.K. Perloff and the *American Journal of Medicine*.)

The latter has revealed contraction abnormalities of the left ventricle in most patients, which is first noted in the posterior free wall behind the mitral valve. But why this portion of the myocardium should be so selectively involved in this particular disorder is not clear. Radionuclide imaging suggests a regional metabolic or blood flow alteration.

Cardiac abnormalities are also very frequently observed in patients with BMD. Despite the milder skeletal muscle involvement in BMD as compared to DMD, cardiac involvement can be detected in more than 60 per cent of patients with BMD. Symptomatic cardiomyopathy is, if anything, more common in BMD compared to DMD, and death from cardiac failure is a well-known complication of this disorder. A few patients with BMD who underwent cardiac transplant have been described. More recently, X-linked dilated cardiomyopathy (XLDCM) has been described as an allelic variant of DMD and BMD. In this condition, in which unusual mutations of the dystrophin gene have been documented, the cardiac muscle is severely affected, with features similar to those observed in DMD and BMD, while the skeletal muscle is virtually spared.

While ECG is a very useful technique for demonstrating the involvement of the cardiac muscle, the correlation with the severity of the cardiomyopathy is relative poor. In clinical practice it is recommended to perform yearly ECG in children. Once an ECG abnormality is noticed, then echocardiographic studies are recommended. If a significant abnormality is detected on echocardiography, most paediatric cardiologists recommend treatment (angiotensin-converting enzyme (ACE) inhibitors, diuretics, low doses of β-blockers), although a large randomized trial of this approach has never been performed. If the echocardiographic abnormalities are mild or the study is normal, repeated echocardiography is indicated. How often echocardiography should be repeated is unclear. In clinical practice we suggest, however, repeating echocardiography every 2 years in non-ambulant DMD patients, or before performing invasive procedures such as spinal surgery. Obviously, if the rate of progression of the observed abnormalities is marked, the echocardiography should be repeated more frequently.

Vascular system

Trophic changes in the skin of the extremities of DMD patients are common, especially in the lower limbs and in the later stages of the disease. These changes include coldness and cyanotic mottling and, on occasion, even scleroderma-like changes. Such changes most probably stem from inactivity, although Duchenne himself even raised the possibility that muscular dystrophy might have a vascular aetiology. Studies that designed to determine if the vascular system is involved in DMD focused, perhaps understandably, on muscle vasculature. Several years ago in Paris, Démos and colleagues (for example, Démos and Maroteaux 1961) measured the circulation time in patients in two ways: arm-to-arm using fluorescein as a marker and arm-to-tongue using sodium dehydrocholate. By subtraction the 'peripheral circulation time' in the upper limb was determined. In boys with DMD, they found this to be above or below the 95 per cent range for normal children of comparable age, and to be significantly reduced in some female carriers. However, there is no defect in the capillary nail bed and, using venous occlusion plethysmography, one of the authors (A.E.) failed to detect any significant changes in total limb blood flow in affected boys at different stages of the disease or in carrier females.

However, more recently, reduced *intramuscular* blood flow has been demonstrated in both the mouse animal model for DMD (the *mdx* mice) and children with DMD. This is believed to be secondary to the absence of nitric oxide synthase (NOS), and hence of nitric oxide, in the skeletal muscle fibres of dystrophin-deficient muscle. As will be discussed later, one of the proteins of the dystrophin-associated glycoprotein complex is neuronal NOS (nNOS). This molecule, physiologically expressed at the periphery of each muscle fibre, is lost from the sarcolemma when dystrophin is also absent. One physiological role of nNOS in skeletal muscle is the production of the NO that mediates the inhibition of sympathetic vasoconstriction in contracting muscle. This ability is defective in the mutant mice that lack the gene encoding nNOS, and also in the *mdx* mouse, in whom nNOS is also secondarily but severely deficient. Recently, a similar defect was confirmed in children with DMD. These observations also suggest another mechanism that might contribute to abnormal smooth muscle function in DMD.

Central nervous system

For some time there was, perhaps understandably, some reluctance to accept that boys with DMD could also be mentally handicapped. After all, this was yet another misfortune for the affected child and his parents to bear. However, much research started in the 1960s confirmed the suspicion of many, first noted in fact by Duchenne, that a proportion of affected boys can have some degree of mental handicap and that, on occasion, this can be severe. It is important to stress that the mental retardation is present in only a minority of patients, and that highly intelligent youngsters with DMD who have satisfactorily completed university degree courses are becoming an increasing reality, in part due to the better opportunity for physically handicapped individuals to attend higher degree studies.

Apart from some degree of intellectual impairment, a deficit of memory and behavioural problems have also been reported.

IQs of affected boys

There have been a great many studies of IQ in affected boys, the results of which were summarized in the previous edition (Emery 1993, p. 116). A total of 721 children were studied in 14 reports, the mean IQ being 82 with 20% having an IQ below 70, and 3% with an IQ below 50 (Table 6.2). There is therefore considerable variation, ranging from those who are severely handicapped to a few with IQs above 130. In general, the overall mean IQ is about one standard deviation below the normal mean. This reduction in IQ is not due to any lack of educational opportunity as an result of their physical disability because it is not found in other diseases with comparable disability, such as severe childhood autosomal recessive muscular dystrophy (SCARMD) or juvenile spinal muscular atrophy. Furthermore, poor educational performance in

Table 6.2 Studies of IQ in boys with DMD ($N = 721$). These figures are based on a large number of published studies (see Emery 1993, p. 116)

IQ	Number of patients (%) with IQ		
Mean	Range IQ	≤70	≤50
82	14–134	19%	3%

DMD is often observed early in life when muscle weakness is relatively slight. Whatever causes the intellectual impairment must also operate at an early stage in development for it is not progressive and does not correlate with duration or severity of the disease. The fact that there is no difference in IQ between affected boys born to carrier mothers and those who are presumed to be the result of new mutations indirectly confirms a specific association between dystrophin mutations and mental retardation and excludes a maternal factor from being responsible for depressing the IQ.

The most likely explanation is that the depression in IQ is another pleiotropic effect of the mutant gene. This is supported by the fact that unaffected sibs have normal intellect, and there is often a good correlation between affected brothers. Several investigators have found a high concordance for intellectual function in families with multiple affected children. It is also our experience that, whenever an index case is severely mentally handicapped (IQ < 50) and has an affected brother, the latter is also severely mentally handicapped. The possibility that there might be bimodality in the distribution of IQ in affected boys was suggested by some earlier studies, but this is refuted by data collected between the 1960s and 1980s (Fig. 6.4).

However, recent correlative data on IQ and site of mutations that take into account the multiple distal and shorter isoforms suggest a complex association. In particular, the severity and frequency of mental retardation increases with a progressive loss of functional distal isoforms. As will be discussed in detail in Chapter 9 and as illustrated in Fig. 6.5, the dystrophin locus generates multiple isoforms from internal promoters located either at the 5' end (the brain, muscle, and cerebellar Purkinje cell isoforms: B, M, and P isoforms) or scattered throughout the gene (see Fig. 6.5). The Dp260 isoform has its first exon in intron 30; Dp140 in intron 45; Dp116 in intron 56; and Dp71 in intron 63 (Fig. 6.5). An out-of-frame deletion of exon 44 will therefore exert its effect on the three 5' full-length isoforms (B, M, and P) and the Dp260 isoform, while the expression of Dp140, Dp116, and Dp71 will be unaffected. In contrast, a deletion extending to exon 50 will also involve the transcription of the Dp140 isoform. A significant contribution of deletions involving the Dp140 isoform to mental retardation has been recently reported

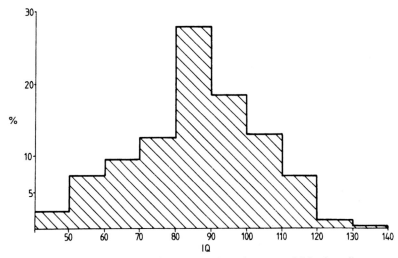

Fig. 6.4 Percentage distribution of IQ in DMD based on 14 published studies.

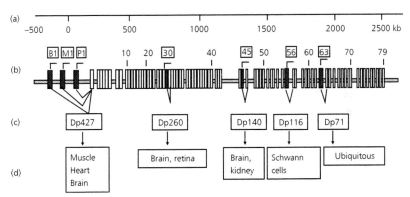

Fig. 6.5 Schematic representation of the dystrophin gene. (a) The size occupied by the dystrophin gene is indicated in kilobases (kb). (b) The locations of the various first exons and promoters are indicated on the top of each of the vertical bars representing the dystrophin exons, while (c) indicates the names of the resulting isoforms. In (b) B1, M1, and P1, respectively, indicate the brain, muscle and Purkinje cell promoters, which are located before exon 2 and encode for three full-length isoforms. The promoter located in intron 30 encodes for the Dp260 isoform, while the one in intron 45 encodes for the Dp140 isoform. the promoters located in introns 56 and 63 are responsible for the transcription of the Dp116 and Dp71 isoforms, respectively. (d) Tissues in which the various isoforms are preferentially expressed.

(Bardoni *et al.* 2000). Finally, mutations that affect all dystrophin isoforms are invariably associated with a severe mental retardation. This has been reported by others and is also the experience of one of the authors (F.M.) who has followed up seven cases with mutations affecting Dp71. Of these, two children never acquired speech and were not testable; the remaining five had moderate to severe mental retardation. In two of these children a diagnosis of autism preceded the diagnosis of muscular dystrophy. For a comprehensive review on dystrophin and brain please refer to Mehler (2000).

Partition of IQ

Several studies have been made to determine what aspect of intellect may be especially affected in DMD by comparing performance and verbal IQs (Table 6.3). In most studies published verbal IQ is more affected, the overall difference from performance IQ being about 5 to 8 points.

The impairment of verbal ability seems to be due to a defect in memory for patterns, numbers, and verbal labels, implying a particular deficit in memory function. Some depression of verbal IQ has also been found in BMD but not in limb girdle or facioscapulohumeral muscular dystrophy.

Relationship between degree of muscle weakness and cognitive involvement

In a study performed over a large number (580) of DMD cases followed at the Hammersmith Hospital, we found that the early motor milestones and the acquisition of ambulation were inversely correlated with mental function, that is, the more severe the mental retardation, the greater the delay in the early motor milestones. On the whole, however, DMD patients with severe mental retardation were not more severely affected than those without mental retardation (personal observation from F.M.). Other studies have, in fact, suggested that DMD children with severe mental retardation seem to be less severely affected. In affected boys with severe mental handicap (IQ < 50), the ages at onset and at becoming confined to a wheelchair were somewhat later (Table 6.4) and the fall in SCK levels with age was less marked.

Table 6.3 Performance (P) and verbal (V) IQ in boys with DMD calculated from data given in eight published studies (full references can be found in Emery 1993, p. 118)

Number of cases	Mean IQ		
	P	V	(P − V)
299	90.65	85.21	+5.44

Table 6.4 Age (years) at onset and at becoming confined to a wheelchair in patients with normal intelligence or with severe mental handicap

Age (years)						*p*	Reference
Normal intelligence			Severe mental handicap				
Number	Mean	SD	Number	Mean	SD		
Age at onset							
15	2.20	0.78	15	2.43	1.03	NS	Emery *et al.* 1979
29	3.64	1.72	10	3.61	2.01	NS	Bortolini and Zatz 1986
Age at becoming chairbound							
12	8.77	1.12	13	9.65	1.60	NS	Emery *et al.* 1979
24	9.49	1.70	11	10.83	1.65	<0.05	Bortolini and Zatz 1986

Behavioural and emotional disturbances

Behavioural and emotional disturbances have been commented upon by a number of investigators and might stem from a sense of failure, frustration, and distress generated by the progressive physical disability. However, in view of the nature of the disorder, it is perhaps surprising that the majority of boys are not emotionally disturbed, and yet they are not. Nevertheless, allowing for age and IQ, boys with DMD do have a higher incidence of emotional disturbances than other physically handicapped children without cerebral involvement, and it is just possible that this too could represent part of the disease. The assessment by one of us (F.M.) of a large series of patients at the Hammersmith Hospital suggests that there might be a small increased risk of epilepsy in children with DMD and BMD. Of 254 boys with these conditions (201 DMD and 53 BMD), eight children (4 DMD and 4 BMD) had confirmed epilepsy, equivalent to a total incidence of 3.14 per cent (with a subgroup incidence of 1.99 per cent in the DMD group and 7.54 per cent in the BMD group). These data suggest that epilepsy may be a rare associated feature in children with muscular dystrophy secondary to dystrophin deficiency but this needs to be confirmed in larger studies.

Neurological investigations

Head circumference appears to be significantly greater than normal but there is no correlation between head size and intellectual performance. However, the rare patients with severe mental retardation and mutations affecting the expression of Dp71 tend to have normal or slightly less than normal head circumference. Electroencephalography (EEG) has been reported as normal in a carefully controlled and blind study by Barwick *et al.* (1965). In some other studies, however, up to a half of the records have been considered abnormal in some non-specific way. Nevertheless, many patients with apparently abnormal EEGs have had normal IQs. In any case, no specific EEG abnormality has been detected in the disease.

Computerized tomography (CT) has been used to study central nervous system involvement. Yoshioka and colleagues in 1980 found evidence of slight cerebral atrophy in two-thirds of the 30 cases they examined, and, the older the patient, the more severe was the atrophy. There were many with a low IQ among those with cerebral atrophy, but in those with apparently normal CT findings only three had a low IQ. Abnormal CT findings therefore seem to be associated with low IQ. Magnetic resonance imaging (MRI), however, has revealed no significant abnormality apart from mild cerebral atrophy in some cases.

From a pathological point of view, two studies have been performed on the brains of children with DMD. IN 1966 Rosman and Kakulas examined the brains of seven DMD cases (two at least of these could have been BMD). In all cases with a mental defect they found microscopic heterotopias in the cerebral cortex. However, in a later more extensive study of 21 cases of classical DMD, Dubowitz and Crome (1969) could detect no gross pathological abnormality. Nevertheless, recent detailed microscopic studies have revealed abnormal dendritic development and arborization, at least in some cases, and this may underlie the intellectual impairment. Dystrophin has been found to be absent in the brain of a boy with DMD. Recent immunocytochemical studies have shown that dystrophin is selectively localized to postsynaptic neurons in cerebral cortex, hippocampus, and cerebellum and colocalizes with γ-aminobutyric acid (GABA)-A receptor subunit clusters in these regions. In the *mdx* mice a marked reduction in the number of clusters immunoreactive for the $\alpha 1$ and $\alpha 2$ GABA subunits was observed in the cerebellum and hippocampus. These data suggest that dystrophin may play an important role in the clustering or stabilization of GABA-A receptors in a subset of central inhibitory synapses (Knuesel *et al.* 1999). The authors concluded that these deficits may be related to the cognitive impairment observed in DMD children.

Though affected boys have normal visual acuity, electroretinography has revealed significant defects in a number of cases. Furthermore, dystrophin has been localized to the outer plexiform layer of the normal retina, and a defect in the retinal isoform in DMD (Dp260; see Fig. 6.5) may account for the observed retinographic changes and also indicates that dystrophin may well play a role in retinal neurotransmission.

Skeletal system

A number of skeletal changes have been observed in DMD. They include progressive narrowing of the shafts of the long bones due to a reduction in the size of the medullary cavity and later thinning of the cortices. Since, at the same time, the head remains more or less the same size, the long bones assume a characteristic 'dumb-bell' appearance (Fig. 6.6). There is often impaired development of the pelvic bones and scapulae, and various skeletal deformities occur including lumbar lordosis, scoliosis, and coxa valga. The bones themselves undergo progressive rarefaction and decalcification beginning at the ends of the long bones.

For a long time these changes were thought to be a direct consequence of a genetic defect, and such terms as 'bone dystrophy' and 'osteomyopathy' were

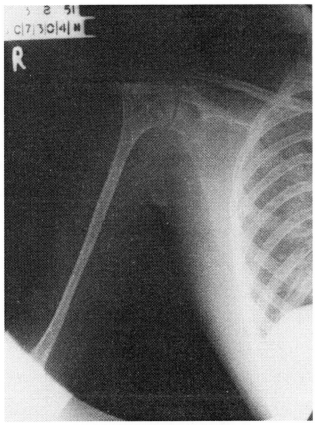

Fig. 6.6 Marked osteoporosis of the humerus in an advanced case of DMD. (Reproduced by kind permission of Lord Walton.)

used. However, it is now quite clear that these same changes can occur in any disorder associated with prolonged immobility. They are not due to an associated genetic factor but to disuse: to the absence of the normal stresses and strains imposed by muscular attachments, and to the adoption of abnormal postures of the body and positions of the limbs as a consequence of muscle weakness and contractures.

Bone densitometry data obtained with dual-energy X-ray absorptiometry (DEXA) scanning have confirmed that children with DMD are significantly osteopenic. Ambulant children with DMD have significantly decreased bone density as early as 5–7 years of age. However, children with other conditions such as limb girdle muscular dystrophy have a similar decrease in bone density suggesting that this problem is secondary to the relative immobility and not a pleiotropic effect of the defective gene.

Other manifestations

Thymus hyperplasia has been reported by several authors, the relevance of which is not at all clear. Puberty can be delayed, hyperoestrogenaemia may occur, and obesity is frequent. However, apart from the study of skeletal muscle, cardiac muscle, and the central nervous system, it has to be admitted that there have been few recent systematic investigations of other systems, organs, or tissues.

With what is known so far, it is possible to construct a simple diagram of the pleiotropic effects of the Duchenne gene (Fig. 6.7). Some of the abnormalities found in the disease relate directly to skeletal, cardiac, and smooth muscle involvement. Others are at present more difficult to relate to the primary protein (dystrophin) defect in the disease.

Summary and conclusions

Most of the clinical features of DMD stem from involvement of skeletal muscle. However, there is increasing evidence that other tissues may also be directly affected by the disease.

Smooth muscle of the gastrointestinal tract and perhaps the bladder may be affected, and there is overwhelming evidence of cardiac muscle involvement, myocardial fibrosis being an important feature. This particularly affects the posterobasal portion of the left ventricle and accounts for the ECG changes of tall R waves in the right praecordial lead that are already evident in the early ambulant phases of the disorder. The vascular system does not appear to be

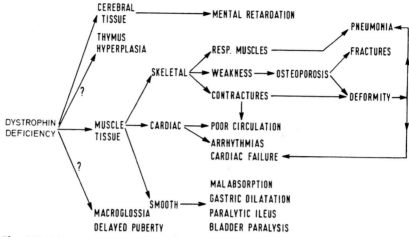

Fig. 6.7 Pleiotropic effects of the Duchenne gene.

significantly affected, although mild reduction of blood flow following exercise related to the deficiency of nitric oxide synthase has now been documented. There is clear evidence of a defect in cerebral function, which is a direct consequence of the genetic defect most obviously expressed in a lowered IQ which, on average, is roughly one standard deviation below the normal mean, verbal IQ being more affected than performance IQ. A pattern of more severe loss of IQ with more distal mutations has been recently suggested. The skeletal system is only secondarily affected by disuse atrophy, and so far there is no convincing evidence that any other tissues or organs are directly affected by the genetic defect.

The various clinical manifestations of DMD are now beginning to be related to the structure and functioning of the dystrophin gene in different tissues. There is much scope for research in relating the phenotype to molecular events in this disease.

References

Bardoni, A., Felisari, G., Sironi, M., Comi, G., Lai, M., Robotti, M., and Bresolin, N. (2000). Loss of Dp140 regulatory sequences is associated with cognitive impairment in dystrophinopathies. *Neuromuscular Disorders* **10** (3), 194–9.

Barwick, D.D., Osselton, J.W., and Walton, J.N. (1965). Electroencephalographic studies in hereditary myopathy. *Journal of Neurology, Neurosurgery and Psychiatry* **28**, 109–14.

Bortolini, E.R. and Zatz, M. (1986). Investigation on genetic heterogeneity in Duchenne muscular dystrophy. *American Journal of Medical Genetics* **24**, 111–17.

Démos, J. and Maroteaux, P. (1961). Mesure des temps de circulation chez 141 sujets normaux par une technique originale. Rôle de la taille de l'enfant sur les temps de circulation de bras à bras. *Revue Française Études Clinique et Biologie* **6**, 773–8.

Dubowitz, V. and Crome, L. (1969). The central nervous system in Duchenne muscular dystrophy. *Brain* **92**, 805–8.

Emery, A.E.H. (1972). Abnormalities of the electrocardiogram in hereditary myopathies. *Journal of Medical Genetics* **9**, 8–12.

Emery, A.E.H. (1993). *Duchenne muscular dystrophy*, 2nd edn. Oxford University Press, Oxford.

Emery, A.E.H., Skinner, R., and Holloway, S. (1979). A study of possible heterogeneity in Duchenne muscular dystrophy. *Clinical Genetics* **15**, 444–9.

Ishikawa, K., Shirato, C., Yotsukura, M., Ishihara, T., Tamura, T., and Inoue, M. (1982). Sequential changes in high frequency notches on QRS complexes in progressive muscular dystrophy of the Duchenne type—a 3-year follow-up study. *Journal of Electrocardiology* **15**, 23–30.

Knuesel, I., Mastrocola, M., Zuellig, R.A., Bornhauser, B., Schaub, M.C., and Fritschy, J.M. (1999). Altered synaptic clustering of GABAA receptors in mice lacking dystrophin (mdx mice). *European Journal of Neuroscience* **11** (12), 4457–62.

Mehler, M.F. (2000). Brain dystrophin, neurogenetics and mental retardation [review]. *Brain Research Reviews* **32** (1), 277–307.

Nadas, A.S. (1963). *Pediatric cardiology*, 2nd edn. Saunders, Philadelphia.

Perloff, J.K., Roberts, W.C., De Leon, A.C., and O'Doherty, D. (1966). The distinctive electrocardiogram of Duchenne's progressive muscular dystrophy. *American Journal of Medicine* **42**, 179–88.

Rosman, N.P. and Kakulas, B.A. (1966). Mental deficiency associated with muscular dystrophy. A neuropathological study. *Neurology* **20**, 329–35.

Yoshioka, M., Okuno, T., Honda, Y., and Nakano, Y. (1980). Central nervous system involvement in progressive muscular dystrophy. *Archives of Disease in Childhood* **55**, 589–94.

Chapter 7

Biochemistry of Duchenne muscular dystrophy

The literature on the biochemistry of muscular dystrophy is overwhelming and many biochemical abnormalities have been reported. It could be argued that, now that the primary defect has been identified in Duchenne muscular dystrophy (DMD) and shown to be a deficiency of muscle dystrophin (Chapter 9), it is irrelevant to approach an understanding of pathogenesis through the findings of conventional biochemistry. We do not share this view but feel that molecular and biochemical studies could complement each other. What has been learned so far concerning biochemical changes in dystrophic muscle and how these relate to the deficiency of dystrophin will doubtless fill in details of how the disease process starts and progresses, and why it affects some muscles more than others. It is also conceivable that the more we know of the detailed pathogenesis of DMD, the more we may understand these processes in other muscular dystrophies. And with such detail it may be possible to better consider a rational approach to any drug therapy.

Selection of material, patients, and controls

One important problem is the selection of appropriate material for study. Muscle is clearly the obvious choice but there is then the problem of assessing the significance of any changes that could be secondary to the disease process. There is also the very serious ethical and practical problem of obtaining material for study and, in practical terms, this is limited to the diagnostic material. The stage of the disease is also important for, clearly, abnormalities found early in the course of the disease are more likely to be closer to the basic biochemical defect.

The choice of appropriate controls is also a problem for the diagnosis is usually established in an affected boy at around 3 to 5 years of age. Appropriate muscle tissue, usually the quadriceps, from a normal boy of this age is not too easily acquired. Also, the use for comparison of muscle tissue from other neuromuscular disorders is questionable unless the research question is to establish whether or not any abnormality is specific to DMD.

Molecular basis

When the gene responsible for a particular disorder can be isolated, cloned, and sequenced, it is possible to see what the gene synthesizes. This has sometimes been referred to as 'reverse genetics' (or positional cloning) for, in the past, it was necessary to start by identifying the product of the defective gene, but now it is possible to identify the mutant gene first and then determine its product. This has been successfully achieved in DMD where the primary genetic defect has been shown to be a deficiency of dystrophin (Chapter 9).

Muscle tissue

There have been many excellent reviews of earlier reported biochemical abnormalities in DMD, and a full reference list of these can be found in the previous edition of the book. It would be impossible to review all the abnormal findings that have been reported, nor would this be valuable. Instead, the discussion will concentrate on those that have been found in early cases of the disease and preferably that have been confirmed in several different laboratories.

It should be pointed out from the beginning that no consistent abnormality in DMD has ever been found in any of the obvious muscle proteins such as myoglobin, actin, myosin, tropomyosin, and troponin. The various biochemical changes that have been observed in affected muscle can be conveniently considered as being the result of wasting, invasion by other tissue elements, and 'dedifferentiation'.

Muscle wasting

As the disease progresses so functioning muscle tissue degenerates, and is gradually replaced by fat and connective tissue. If the results are expressed in terms of total muscle weight then particular constituents may appear to be reduced when, in fact, the levels in functioning muscle tissue may be normal. A solution to this problem is to express results in terms of some specific reference base. In the past this has been total protein or, better still, non-collagen protein, which corresponds to that fraction of the total muscle protein that is soluble in dilute alkali. In health the amount of non-collagen protein (expressed as non-collagen nitrogen) is roughly the same in different skeletal muscles (Table 7.1) and, at least in later childhood and young adulthood, it is not significantly affected by age or sex. Non-collagen protein represents over 90 per cent of the total protein of normal muscle but it may be less than 50 per cent in severely affected dystrophic muscle.

Myosin or some similar contractile protein has also been recommended as a reference base. Whereas fibroblasts, macrophages, lipocytes, and other cells

Table 7.1 Non-collagen nitrogen (NCN) expressed as mg (g wet weight)$^{-1}$, in various normal human skeletal muscles (unpublished data)

Muscle	Number	NCN	
		Mean	SD
Rectus abdominis	20	23.3	6.2
Gastrocnemius	8	26.7	5.5
Deltoid	6	20.7	2.7
Pectoralis major	10	23.9	5.6
Miscellaneous*	9	24.0	3.6
Total	53	23.7	5.3

* Quadriceps (3); sternomastoid (2); sartorius (1); transversalis (1); diaphragm (1); latissimus dorsi (1).

present in dystrophic tissue might contribute to non-collagen protein, they would not affect the myosin content. As would be expected, as dystrophic muscle degenerates so its myosin content decreases. When levels of ATP and creatine phosphate are expressed in terms of myosin they are no different from normal. This result is in stark contrast to several earlier studies that reported reduced levels using non-collagen protein as the reference base. Normal levels of ATP have also been confirmed by the technique of nuclear magnetic resonance (NMR). The fact that ATP levels are normal has important implications. It means that energy stores for muscle contraction are adequate, at least early in the course of the disease, and therefore this is not the cause of muscle weakness. The latter seems more likely to be a reflection of the loss of muscle fibres due to their degeneration.

However, studies using NMR spectroscopy seem to indicate that creatine phosphate may be reduced (Fig. 7.1).

As the amount of functioning muscle tissue decreases, this has several other consequences. Occasionally, the glucose tolerance curve may be mildly abnormal, due to an inadequate disposal of glucose associated with the reduced muscle mass, and plasma free fatty acids may be raised. Glucose and lipid metabolism have been studied in detail and the abnormal energy metabolism observed is attributed to either calorie shortage or, more probably, muscle degeneration. More importantly, changes occur in creatine and creatinine metabolism, changes that have also been recognized for many years. Creatine is largely synthesized in the liver and is delivered to the skeletal muscle where it is converted to creatinine, which readily diffuses into the circulation and is excreted in the urine. In fact, the amount of creatinine excreted each day by any individual is remarkably constant and is roughly proportional to the total body muscle mass.

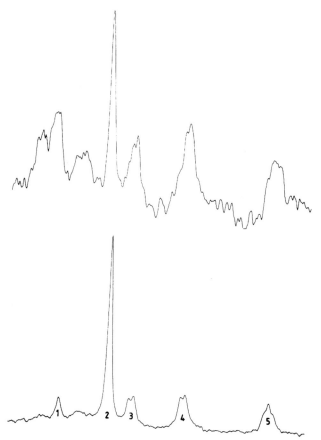

Fig. 7.1 Magnetic resonance spectra of gastrocnemius muscle in a control (below), and a 15-year-old boy with DMD (above). In the affected boy there is a significant increase in intracellular pH (normal 7.01, affected 7.28) and an apparent reduction in the ratio of creatine phosphate to inorganic phosphate. Peaks: 1, inorganic phosphate; 2, creatine phosphate; 3–5, ATP. (Reproduced by kind permission of Dr S.P. Frostick.)

In general terms, as muscle wastes from whatever cause, so the level of creatine in the plasma and especially the urine will increase, and the amount of creatinine in the urine will decrease. These changes, however, appear to be somewhat removed from the basic defect in dystrophy, not only because they are not specific, but also because no abnormalities in creatine and creatinine excretion occur in female carriers of the disease unless they have significant muscle weakness (Emery 1963). Of 10 female carriers investigated, in only one, who was a manifesting carrier with marked muscle weakness, was the creatine/creatinine ratio abnormally high (Fig. 7.2).

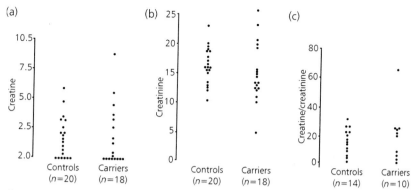

Fig. 7.2 The urinary excretion of (a) creatine, (b) creatinine (mg kg^{-1} 24 h^{-1}), and (c) ratio of creatine/creatinine ($\times$100) in healthy women and DMD carriers. (Unpublished data.)

As skeletal muscle degenerates, various breakdown products will be released and appear in the urine. For example, 3-methylhistidine is a known constituent of both actin and myosin, and, as muscle breaks down, the concentration in muscle decreases, and, when expressed in terms of creatinine, the urinary excretion increases. In fact, the urinary excretion of 3-methylhistidine is an excellent measurement of myofibrillar protein catabolism. Thus, while creatinine excretion may be taken as an index of total muscle mass, 3-methylhistidine excretion is an index of muscle breakdown.

Carnitine is largely synthesized in the liver and kidneys and is subsequently taken up by cardiac and skeletal muscle. As muscle breaks down so carnitine is released and concentrations in dystrophic muscle are significantly reduced. Since carnitine is an important co-factor in fatty acid oxidation, the reduction in muscle carnitine might also explain the accumulation of long-chain fatty acid derivatives in this tissue.

Finally, although there is no doubt that many proteins are lost from dystrophic muscle, there is also evidence that some substances may actually enter affected muscle fibres. Experimentally, ingress of horseradish peroxidase (molecular weight (MW), 40 000 Da), and Procion yellow (MW 674 Da) have been demonstrated, and evidence suggests that calcium, IgG, complement, and albumin enter affected muscle fibres (see Chapter 10). Of particular interest is the finding that calcium and albumin enter fibres lacking dystrophin in female carriers of X-linked dystrophy. This has important implications for pathogenesis and will be discussed later (Chapter 10).

The abnormal plasma membrane permeability in dystrophin-deficient muscle can also be assessed *in vivo* in the animal models of muscular dystrophy using tracer molecules such as Evans Blue. This low molecular weight diazo dye, does not cross into skeletal muscle fibres in normal mice. In contrast, *mdx* mice showed significant Evans blue accumulation in skeletal muscle fibres. The Evans blue accumulation is significantly increased by strenuous physical exercise, providing some evidence for the exercise-induced damage of muscle fibres (Straub *et al.* 1997).

More recently, an albumin-targeted contrast agent (MS-325) was used *in vivo* to study sarcolemmal integrity of *mdx* mice by MRI. Intravenously injected MS-325 does not enter skeletal muscle of normal mice. However, *mdx* mice showed significant accumulation of MS-325 in skeletal muscle. The results indicate that it is possible to use this non-invasive technique for evaluating the localization and severity of skeletal muscle damage in muscular dystrophy.

Enzyme changes in dystrophic muscle

There is general agreement that glycolysis as well as the activities of most individual glycolytic enzymes is reduced in muscle from DMD patients as well as in several other dystrophies. Ellis's (1980) detailed studies indicate that, in dystrophic muscle, fructose is incorporated into the glycogen pathway at the expense of glucose and this results in increased lipogenesis. Fatty acid oxidation is also reduced but, again, this is not specific to DMD.

A great many individual enzymes have been studied in muscle tissue from patients with DMD. In those instances where enzyme levels have been expressed in terms of non-collagen protein and studies made specifically on DMD, some general conclusions can be made. The level of activity of some enzymes appears to be normal, at least in the early stages of the disease (Table 7.2).

Other enzymes, however, have reduced activity (Table 7.3), in some cases even from very early on in the disease process as in the case of AMP deaminase. Interestingly, a deficiency of the erythrocyte form of phosphofructokinase is not associated with muscle disease but results in a non-spherocytic haemolytic anaemia.

The reduced activity of these various enzymes is probably largely the result of efflux from diseased muscle fibres though this cannot be the entire story. Thus, adenylate kinase, which has a relatively low molecular weight (21 000 Da), is reduced in affected muscle but is not increased in serum (Chapter 4) and this is also true of AMP deaminase. On the other hand, the aminotransferases are not significantly reduced in affected muscle but are increased in serum. Finally, acyl phosphatase is one of the smallest enzyme molecules known (9 400 Da) and is abundant in skeletal muscle, largely in the soluble sarcoplasm, yet there is apparently normal activity in affected muscle. The explanation for these apparent contradictions may lie in the relative rates of synthesis

Table 7.2 Enzymes with normal activity in skeletal muscle tissue in DMD

Aminotransferases (GPT, GOT)
Succinic dehydrogenase
Hexokinase
Phosphohexose isomerase
Aconitase
Cytochrome oxidase
Alkaline phosphatase
Acyl phosphatase
Fructose 1,6-diphosphatase
Lysolecithin phospholipase
Superoxide dismutase
Methylthioadenosine nucleosidase
Adenylosuccinase
Monamine oxidase
Glyoxalase II

Table 7.3 Enzymes with reduced activity in skeletal muscle tissue in DMD

Phosphoglucomutase
Phosphofructokinase
Aldolase
Triosephosphate isomerase
Phosphoglyceraldehyde dehydrogenase
Phosphoglycerate kinase
Enolase
Pyruvate kinase
Lactate dehydrogenase
Fumarase
Glycogen phosphorylase
Glycogen synthetase
Creatine kinase
AMP deaminase
Adenylate kinase

(perhaps influenced to some extent by physical activity) versus destruction of different enzymes in affected muscle fibres, as well as their clearance rates from plasma. So far, however, very little is known of the relative importance of these different factors for individual enzymes.

Finally, and perhaps more interestingly, the activity of some enzymes is actually increased in DMD (Table 7.4). These changes are attributable to the invasion of affected muscle by macrophages and fibroblasts, as well as to the necrosis of affected muscle fibres. Macrophages and fibroblasts are known to contain several nicotinamide-adenine dinucleotide phosphate (NADP)-linked dehydrogenases (glucose-6-phosphate dehydrogenase, 6-phosphogluconate dehydrogenase, isocitrate dehydrogenase, and malate dehydrogenase), and other enzymes such as 5'-nucleotidase and ribonuclease. These cells also contain a number of proteases, including cathepsins, lysosomal acid hydrolases, and calcium-activated proteases, which are all increased in dystrophic muscle. These enzymes attack and break down muscle protein and their increase is probably also an adaptive response of the muscle fibre to its degeneration and necrosis.

It should be noted, however, that this division into enzymes that are normal, reduced, or increased in dystrophic muscle, although convenient, is somewhat arbitrary because it often depends at what stage in the disease process the assays are carried out. In almost all cases activity is normal at the beginning and abnormally low or high levels are found only later in the course of the disease. But some, such as acyl phosphatase, seem to remain at more or less normal levels right until the very late stages of the disease.

Table 7.4 Enzymes with increased activity in skeletal muscle tissue in DMD

Glucose-6-phosphate dehydrogenase
6-Phosphogluconate dehydrogenase
Isocitrate dehydrogenase
Malate dehydrogenase
5'-Nucleotidase
Ribonuclease
Glutathione reductase
Prote(in)ases
Carnitine palmityltransferase
Lipid peroxidation
Phosphodiesterases

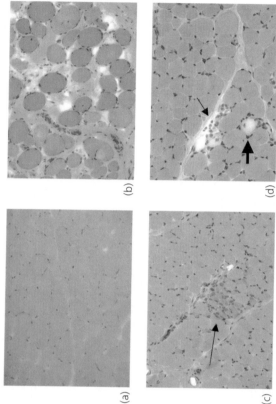

Plate 2 (a) Normal muscle. (b) Duchenne muscle with hypercontracted fibres, abundant connective tissue, fat, and internal nuclei. (c) Duchenne muscle with cluster of basophilic regenerating fibres (arrow) and only mild fibrosis. (d) Duchenne muscle showing a small cluster of necrotic fibres (small arrows) and an isolated one (big arrow). See Figure 4.6.

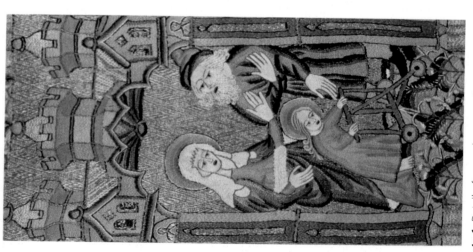

Plate 1 Detail of an orphery on a fourteenth century dalmatic in The Burrell Collection, Glasgow. See frontispiece.

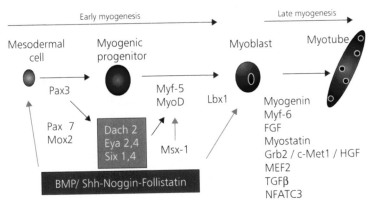

Plate 3 The site of action of myogenic factors during muscle development. See Figure 7.7.

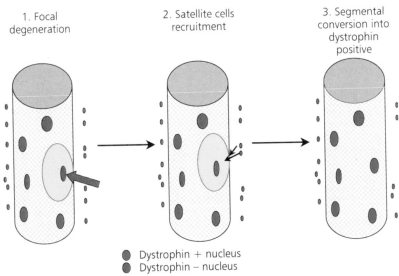

● Dystrophin + nucleus
● Dystrophin − nucleus

Plate 4 The model of biochemical normalization. See Figure 11.2.

Membrane enzymes

Many muscle enzymes are free in the sarcoplasm but some are attached to membranes, such as the sarcoplasmic reticulum. The latter include adenylate cyclase, guanylate cyclase, and Ca^{2+}-, $(Na^+ + K^+)$-, and Mg^{2+}-ATPases. Until fairly recently, enzyme studies have been limited to whole muscle homogenates, which, at least later in the disease, are contaminated by extraneous adipose and connective tissue. It has, therefore, not been possible to study the activity in isolation of those enzymes that are attached specifically to muscle membranes. To circumvent this problem minimally affected muscle should be studied, and the technique of using 'skinned fibres' has been developed. In these preparations the surface membrane of the muscle fibre is removed mechanically or disrupted chemically. Using these techniques it seems that, in the early stages of the disease, the sarcoplasmic reticulum and contractile protein functions are normal as is calcium uptake by the sarcoplasmic reticulum. The study of skinned fibres has also shown that, in DMD, despite the deficiency of dystrophin, these contract normally and therefore the myofibrils must themselves be intrinsically normal.

'Dedifferentiation'

A number of observations indicate that in many ways dystrophic muscle resembles fetal muscle for which the term 'dedifferentiation' has sometimes been used. Firstly, it is less easy to distinguish different histochemical fibre types in dystrophic muscle, which is also a feature of fetal muscle (Fig. 7.3) even at term. Secondly, certain phospholipid changes in dystrophic muscle (more sphingomyelin, less lecithin plus choline plasmalogen, and more total cholesterol) are very similar to those found in fetal muscle. Thirdly, fetal myosins are found in muscle from patients with DMD and spinal muscular atrophy. Fourthly, another fetal isoform of muscle protein re-expressed in regenerating muscle is cardiac troponin-T.

Finally, and most intriguingly, the isoenzyme patterns of dystrophic muscle resemble those of fetal muscle rather than adult muscle. This was first shown in the case of lactate dehydrogenase (LDH). This enzyme is composed of five isoenzymes, each being formed by the tetrameric association of two subunits, synthesized by two separate genes, referred to as M and H (Fig. 7.4). The M subunit predominates in adult skeletal muscle and the H subunit in cardiac muscle.

On electrophoresis the most rapidly migrating isoenzyme LDH-1 has the composition H_4, LDH-2 $= H_3M$, LDH-3 $= H_2$, M_2, LDH-4 $= HM_3$, and LDH-5 $= M_4$. The amounts and proportions of the M and H subunits (LDH-M, LDH-H) can be determined in a number of ways. The proportions of LDH-M and LDH-H in some normal skeletal muscles are given in Table 7.5.

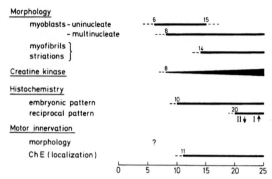

Fig. 7.3 Times (weeks of gestation) at which various aspects of muscle development become apparent. ChE, Choline esterase. (Data from various sources.)

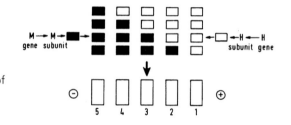

Fig. 7.4 The formation of the five isoenzymes of lactate dehydrogenase.

Table 7.5 Proportions (%) of LDH-M and LDH-H in various normal skeletal muscles (unpublished data)

Muscle	Number	Proportion (%)	
		LDH-M	LDH-H
Rectus abdominis	5	87.0	13.0
Diaphragm	1	89.2	10.8
Gastrocnemius	3	86.7	13.3
Quadriceps	1	89.6	10.4
Latissimus dorsi	1	87.4	12.6
Pectoralis major	6	87.9	12.1
Deltoid	2	95.6	4.4
Soleus	2	67.1	32.9

Although there are some variations in different skeletal muscles, LDH-M clearly predominates. However, in fetal skeletal muscle LDH-H predominates, and the isoenzyme pattern resembles that seen in DMD even in the preclinical phase (Fig. 7.5). It may be that the normal adult pattern is never attained, in which case the term 'dedifferentiation' is hardly appropriate. Incidentally, there does not appear to be a complete absence of LDH-5 in all cases of DMD. A reduction in LDH-M is also found in some female carriers but the change is not specific to DMD but is also found in a number of other neuromuscular disorders. Analogous changes in isoenzyme patterns have also been reported for creatine kinase, aldolase, isocitrate dehydrogenase, malate dehydrogenase, adenylate kinase, and enolase.

The implication of these various findings is that dystrophic muscle synthesizes polypeptides not normally produced postnatally and that these changes are presumably a result of regenerative activity: newly synthesized peptides reflecting the activity of genes normally active only during fetal development. The enzyme hypoxanthine-guanine phosphoribosyltransferase is significantly increased in muscle in patients with DMD even from the age of 2, and this has been interpreted as being a means of enhancing increased protein synthesis and regenerative activity. Finally, using immunohistochemical techniques, the

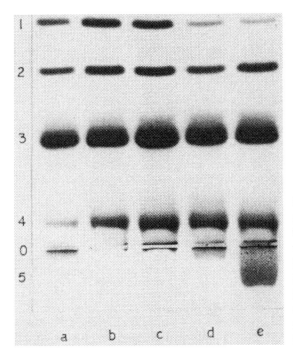

Fig. 7.5 LDH isoenzyme patterns in muscle extracts from: (a) 3-year-old boy with preclinical DMD; (b) 400 g fetus; (c) 7-month stillbirth; (d) neonate; (e) 3-month-old normal infant. 0 is the origin and the anode is at the top.

re-expression of fetal-specific myosins has also been localized to regenerating fibres in DMD.

Despite these detailed studies, the mechanism of progressive muscle fibre necrosis in dystrophin-deficient muscular dystrophies is completely unknown. The answer to the fundamental question as to whether a deficit of muscle energy production plays a relevant role in the cascade of events starting with dystrophin deficiency and ending with muscle fibre degeneration is also not known. Magnetic resonance spectroscopy (MRS) data obtained *in vivo* have added further evidence suggesting that specific and significant metabolic abnormalities can be identified in the dystrophin-deficient skeletal muscle. Furthermore, recent gene profiling data obtained from the muscle of DMD children and *mdx* mice provide additional evidence of the importance of the secondary metabolic imbalance observed in the dystrophin-deficient muscle. In view of the many biochemical and muscle enzyme changes that have been well documented in DMD for some years, it is, of course, not at all surprising that gene profiling studies have found the transcription levels of many genes to be altered. These latter data will be discussed in detail in Chapter 10.

Regarding MRS studies, skeletal muscle oxidative and non-oxidative energy production have been analysed both in DMD and Becker muscular dystrophy (BMD) muscle *in vivo* (Lodi *et al.* 1999). The main findings are that, following aerobic exercise, the dystrophin-deficient muscle acidifies less than normally. In particular, the cytosolic pH at the end of exercise is significantly higher in patients compared to controls. The rate of proton efflux from muscle fibres of patients is similar to that of controls and this points towards a deficit in glycolytic lactate production as a cause of higher end-exercise cytosolic pH in patients. In these patients proton efflux measured during the initial part of post-exercise recovery was not different from that of controls indicating that reduced lactate production through glycolysis is the more likely explanation for the reduced acidification. The fact that this is manifest only in the later stages of the exercise suggests that this abnormality lies in the utilization of glucose rather than glycogen, and thus in the glucose transport and/or hexokinase steps. The interpretation of these findings *in vivo* as being due to a glycolytic defect is consistent with a number of observations *in vitro* of altered glucose metabolism in dystrophin-deficient muscle. The glucose transporter GLUT4, which co-localizes with dystrophin and other dystrophin-associated proteins, including neuronal nitric oxide synthase (nNOS) on the inner sarcolemmal membrane, is reduced in the diaphragm and heart of *mdx* mice to approximately 50 per cent of the normal value. Furthermore, nNOS is also significantly decreased in dystrophin-deficient skeletal muscle, and this might contribute to the deficit in glycolytic lactate production in dystrophin-deficient muscle, as nNOS increases the rate of glucose transport and metabolism in skeletal muscle.

Whether and how the glycolytic deficit in dystrophin-deficient muscle contributes to fibre necrosis is difficult to establish. It is, however, possible that, during exercise, the glycolytic deficit may be responsible for greater ionic imbalance and that this may be related to chronic skeletal muscle injury.

Cultured myoblasts

The study of myoblasts in tissue culture, free from all the possible confounding effects of extraneous factors, would seem to offer the ideal system for studying DMD. Unfortunately, there are technical difficulties to be overcome in this approach, not least of which is the presence of other cell types (mostly fibroblasts) that 'contaminate' such cultures. This is particularly a problem with primary explants where the biopsy material is first freed of any obvious fat and connective tissue, and then small fragments, about 1 mm in size, are grown in culture vessels with appropriate nutrient medium, usually enriched with chick embryo extract or fetal calf serum. To avoid problems of possible contamination with fibroblasts, cellular outgrowths from explants can be dissociated and the dissociated cells then transferred to secondary monolayer cultures, a procedure that can be repeated. In this way we chose to study fetal muscle in which fibroblast contamination is minimal in any event (Fig. 7.6). A dissociation technique coupled with special culture conditions can also be used, which ensures that growth of myoblasts is encouraged at the expense of other cell types.

As a further refinement, clonal cultures can be set up whereby the progeny of single myoblasts can be studied. Finally, muscle-nerve co-cultures (for example, DMD muscle and rodent spinal cord) can be used to study the possible effects of innervation *in vitro*.

Whether muscle is cultured aneurally or innervated, no gross morphological abnormalities are evident in DMD. Detailed scanning electron microscopic studies, however, have revealed changes in cell surface morphology, which could explain the low adhesiveness and delayed fusion of dystrophic myoblasts in culture, and these abnormalities are expressed maximally after myoblast fusion. Some reported biochemical abnormalities have been interpreted as indicating that dystrophic muscle in culture reaches a lesser degree of maturity than normal muscle. For example, in dystrophic muscle culture creatine kinase BB isoenzyme is significantly increased (and the CK MM decreased), although this is not specific to DMD. The protein degradation rate in cultured Duchenne muscle cells is normal, which supports the idea that the loss of contractile muscle proteins in the disease is largely the result of reduced synthesis rather than increased degradation.

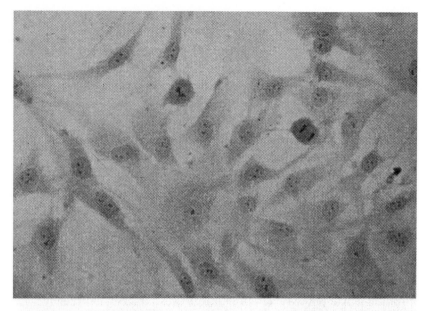

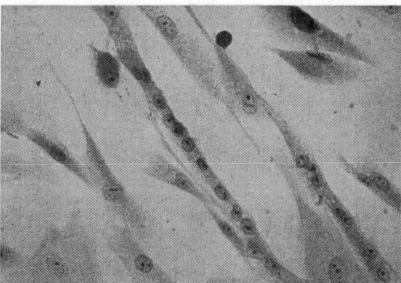

Fig. 7.6 Fetal muscle in tissue culture. (Above) Dividing uninucleate myoblasts. (Below) Fusion of myoblasts to form multinucleate myotubes.

With regard to the expression of dystrophin in cultured muscle, normally it is not demonstrable in undifferentiated myoblasts but appears only after myoblast fusion to form myotubes. We have shown that dystrophin is apparent already after 4 days in fusion media, although not all desmin-positive cells are also dystrophin-positive, confirming that desmin is a protein expressed much earlier during development. Dystrophin appears first in circumscribed areas in the sarcoplasm but later in more mature myotubes it appears predominantly at the sarcolemma. Since these observations have been made with cultured aneural muscle and in the absence of 'trophic' nerve factors, the expression of dystrophin *per se* does not require innervation. As expected in cultured Duchenne muscle, dystrophin is virtually absent, even in mature myotubes. We documented a positive 'revertant' myotube in fetal muscle that was otherwise entirely dystrophin-negative. Regarding clonal myogenic cell cultures from DMD carriers, , some clones express dystrophin whereas others do not. Cultured BMD muscle expresses dystrophin with an expected abnormal molecular weight.

What light do these various studies throw on the pathogenesis of DMD? Perhaps one of the most interesting findings is an increase in intracellular calcium in aneurally cultured dystrophic muscle at a time when dystrophin would be expressed in normal tissue. However, the relationship between innervation, the expression of dystrophin, and subsequent intracellular events is complex. Muscle development both *in vitro* and *in vivo* involves the interplay of a number of myogenic factors as well as innervation (Fig. 7.7).

The interactions between these factors and dystrophin expression might be crucial in determining the full expression of dystrophy in cultured cells. As Valerie Askanas (personal communication) postulated:

> . . . even though there is dystrophin deficiency in cultured Duchenne muscle, only some aspects of the abnormal phenotype, namely calcium accumulation (aneural cultures) and decreased CK-MM (innervated cultures), are expressed. It is possible that more advanced maturation of muscle is required for the full expression of an abnormal phenotype in Duchenne muscle in culture, which would be similar to the situation occurring *in vivo* . . .'.

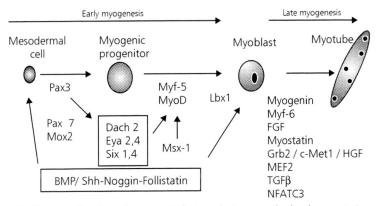

Fig. 7.7 The site of action of myogenic factors during muscle development. See colour plate section in the centre of this book.

Another important recent finding relates to the replicative ageing of myogenic cells (satellite cells) due to increased myofibre turnover. This has been correlated with progressive telomere reduction, which, by limiting the proliferative capacity of dystrophic human myoblasts, also limits their ability to be genetically modified and used for myoblast transplantation. However, not all studies on telomere length measurements in dystrophic tissue have been consistent. If the findings of replicative ageing are confirmed, it could possibly be 'treated' by telomerase gene delivery.

Cultured fibroblasts

The growth, behaviour, morphology, and biochemistry of skin fibroblasts in tissue culture from DMD patients have been studied extensively. Unfortunately, some earlier observations have either not been corroborated subsequently, or have not been repeated and it is often difficult to assess the relevance of an isolated finding. Recently, the possibility that DMD fibroblasts might exert a paracrine effect by diffusible factors was suggested by experiments on Duchenne fibroblast/normal myoblast co-cultures. These studies also identified altered expression of IGF-binding proteins mRNA, with upregulation of IGFBP-5 and downregulation of IGFBP-3 mRNA. The relevance of these findings is currently difficult to interpret in view of the virtual lack of dystrophin gene expression in fibroblasts. Indeed, only very low levels of 'illegitimate' transcription of dystrophin have been demonstrated in skin fibroblasts. The amounts of transcript synthesized are so small that their physiological role is questionable.

Serum

Most studies have concentrated on the levels of various muscle enzymes in the serum of DMD patients. Elevated levels of most enzymes can be accounted for by their relative abundance in muscle tissue as compared with serum, and their release from dystrophic muscle into the circulation. It has been suggested that enzymes may also be released from other organs, including the liver, but the evidence is not very convincing. Certainly the characteristic liver enzymes, γ-glutamyltransferase and sorbitol dehydrogenase, are normal. It is interesting to note that a significant elevation of transaminases is regularly found in DMD, and in the past it was not unusual in this context for several presymptomatic children with DMD or BMD to be extensively investigated for possible liver disease before a neuromuscular disease was suspected.

A large number of studies were performed in the 1960s and 1970s on the possibility that circulating 'toxins' might contribute to pathogenesis of muscular dystrophy. Many of these observations were controversial at the time and have not been repeated since.

Urine

As in the case of serum, no abnormal metabolites have been detected in urine specifically in DMD. The changes in urinary composition that have been observed can all be explained on the basis of the release of various breakdown products from degenerating muscle into the circulation and then excretion in the urine. As we have seen, the urinary excretion of creatine is increased, whereas the excretion of creatinine is decreased so that the ratio of creatine to creatinine in the urine is significantly increased.

Breakdown products excreted in increased amounts in urine, when expressed in terms of creatinine, include carnitine, various amino acids, and 3-methylhistidine. The aminoaciduria in DMD is generalized with no consistent pattern (plasma amino acid levels are normal). Frank myoglobinuria is not normally associated with DMD. However, we have observed a few instances of spontaneous myoglobinuria in toddlers with DMD.

None of these changes in urinary composition are specific to DMD but may be found in any neuromuscular disorder in which muscle breakdown occurs. The increased urinary excretion of dimethylarginines in muscular dystrophy, however, has a different origin. N^G, N^G-Dimethylarginine is mainly located in cell nuclei as a component of non-histone nuclear protein and its increased excretion reflects myosin turnover in muscle regenerating from satellite cells. It is, therefore, an index of regenerative activity and could be a useful parameter for assessing the value of any proposed therapy.

Animal models

Various neuromuscular disorders have been described in many animals including mink, sheep, duck, cow, dog, cat hamster, and chicken, but only a few of these have turned out to be associated with secondary dystrophin deficiency. These are the dystrophic mouse *mdx*, the dystrophic dog, and the dystrophic cat and will be discussed below. Of these, only the clinical picture of the dog model has significant resemblance to the human disease.

Muscular dystrophy in the mouse

In 1984 a spontaneous dystrophin mutant was identified in the C57BL/10 inbred strain, referred to as *mdx*. Points of similarity with DMD are the X-linked mode of inheritance, elevated serum levels of creatine kinase and pyruvate kinase, primary involvement of skeletal muscle, and an absence of muscle dystrophin (human and mouse dystrophins are very similar). But there are significant differences from the human disease. The first and most important point is the lack of significant weakness in the *mdx* mice. Indeed, the *mdx* mouse strain was identified by the chance finding of elevated SCK and not because of significant muscle weakness. Recent studies suggest, however, that aged *mdx* mice do show some degree of muscle weakness, and might have shorter life span. Also, the muscle histology is different because, though muscle degeneration is evident early on, subsequently regeneration occurs, the regenerated fibres remaining centrally nucleated (Fig. 7.8). Interestingly, the muscle degeneration starts at 2–3 weeks of age, affecting first the axial and proximal muscles and extending subsequently to the distal muscles. The regeneration is, however, very efficient and the loss of muscle fibres and progressive fibrosis very limited. This is the main reason for affected mice remaining essentially normal with no obvious weakness. The diaphragm is the only muscle to show progressive degeneration, although significant fibrosis has been demonstrated in various muscles in the old mice.

The molecular basis of the disorder in the *mdx* is a point mutation causing a stop codon in exon 23 of the dystrophin gene. More recently, various chemical-induced mutants have been generated with point mutations in different parts of the gene, some of which affect also the 3′ distal isoforms of dystrophin (for a review see Noguchi and Hayashi 2001).

Although the *mdx* mouse provides a good model for some aspects of DMD, the most intriguing question it poses is why is the disease much milder than the human equivalent? An answer to this question could be of considerable significance in understanding the cause of progressive weakness in the human disease.

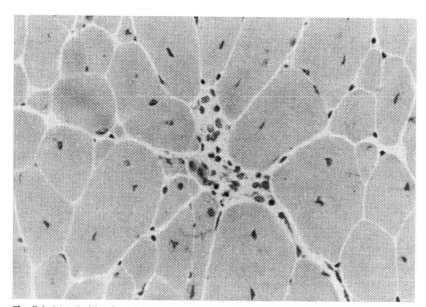

Fig. 7.8 Muscle histology in mouse mutant *mdx*. Note the variation in fibre size and the preponderance of central nuclei. (Haematoxylin and eosin.)

Muscular dystrophy in the cat

Dystrophin deficiency has also been described in male cats in which the histopathology is remarkable and shows muscle hypertrophy with progressive accumulation of calcium. Clinically, it seems unique in that diaphragmatic and glossal hypertrophy are predominant features, though the latter is not uncommon in DMD. The glossal hypertrophy can be severe to the point that the affected cat can die because of malnutrition. Some affected cats can also develop severe muscle stiffness.

In the dystrophic cat, like the *mdx* mouse but unlike the human disease and the dystrophic dog, there is no progressive loss of muscle fibres, no progressive fibrosis, and no progressive weakness despite the deficiency of dystrophin. The molecular basis for the dystrophin deficiency in these cats is a deletion of the muscle promoter.

Muscular dystrophy in the dog

Breeds of dog with an X-linked muscular dystrophy associated with a reduction or absence of dystrophin (which in the dog is identical to that in humans) are found in the golden retriever, the wire-haired fox terrier, the Rottweiler, and the German short-haired pointer. In many ways these dystrophies are more comparable to DMD because the muscle pathology is more-or-less identical to the human disease, and muscle weakness is progressive with the later development of limb contractures. In the retriever, but not the fox terrier, occasional dystrophin-positive fibres occur as in DMD.

The molecular basis for the disorder in the golden retriever model is a point mutation within the splice site of intron 6 of the dystrophin gene, causing a deletion of exon 7 from the transcript with loss of the open reading frame. So far, these breeds are the best animal models of the human disease and could provide excellent subjects for studying the effects of any therapeutic approaches to the disease. Both the Rottweiler and the German short-haired pointer have more severe clinical and pathological features than the golden retrievers and also suffer from dilated cardiomyopathy.

The study of the reasons for these species differences could be very revealing and help our understanding of the pathogenesis of the human disorder.

Summary and conclusions

Many biochemical abnormalities have been found in DMD. Abnormal findings are likely to be relevant to pathogenesis only when they relate specifically to DMD and occur in the *very early* stages of the disease process before there is any significant muscle wasting and weakness.

Muscle tissue has been studied the most, and the observed biochemical changes are conveniently considered as being the consequence of three main processes. Firstly, there are those changes that result from wasting and degeneration—these include the reduction in muscle myosin, carnitine, and most glycolytic enzymes. Secondly, there are changes attributable to the invasion of affected muscle by macrophages, lymphocytes, and fibroblasts as well as to the necrosis of affected muscle fibres. These include the increase in enzymes present in fibroblasts and macrophages (such as NADP-linked dehydrogenases), proteases (cathepsins, lysosomal acid hydrolases, and calcium-activated proteases), and immune-related proteins and HLA antigens. Thirdly, in many ways dystrophic muscle resembles fetal muscle (histochemically, and lipid, myosin, and isoenzyme patterns) for which the term 'dedifferentiation' has sometimes been used. The balance of evidence indicates that mitochondrial oxidation, sarcoplasmic reticulum, and contractile protein functions are essentially normal, at least in the *early stages* of the disease. However, a deficiency in glucose utilization, possibly linked to the absence of dystrophin and the secondary deficiency of GLUT4, has been demonstrated using MRS.

The results of studies on cultured dystrophic myoblasts have shown that there is a deficiency of dystrophin but only some aspects of the abnormal phenotype are expressed by these cells in culture.

So far, the best animal models of DMD are the *mdx* mouse and certain breeds of golden retriever. In all these models the disease is X-linked and associated with a deficiency of muscle dystrophin. However, the disease is only progressive in the dog models, which could therefore provide the best animal models for therapeutic trials.

References

Ellis, D.A. (1980). Intermediary metabolism of muscle in Duchenne muscular dystrophy. *British Medical Bulletin* **36**, 165–1.

Emery, A.E.H. (1963). Clinical manifestations in two carriers of Duchenne muscular dystrophy. *Lancet* **i**, 1126–8.

Lodi, R., Kemp, G.J., Muntoni, F., Thompson, C.H., Rae, C., Taylor, J., Styles, P., and Taylor, D.J. (1999). Reduced cytosolic acidification during exercise suggests defective glycolytic activity in skeletal muscle of patients with Becker muscular dystrophy—an *in vivo* P-31 magnetic resonance spectroscopy study. *Brain* **122**, 121–30.

Noguchi, S. and Hayashi, Y.K. (2001). Animal models of muscular dystrophy. In *The muscular dystrophies* (ed. A.E.H. Emery), pp 297–309. Oxford University Press, Oxford.

Straub, V., Rafael, J.A., Chamberlain, J.S., and Campbell, K.P. (1997). Animal models for muscular dystrophy show different patterns of sarcolemmal disruption. *Journal of Cell Biology* **139** (2), 375–85.

Straub, V., Donahue, K.M., Allamand, V., Davisson, R.L., Kim, Y.R., and Campbell, K.P. (2000). Contrast agent-enhanced magnetic resonance imaging of skeletal muscle damage in animal models of muscular dystrophy. *Magnetic Resonance Medicine* **44** (4), 655–9.

Chapter 8

Genetics

The familial nature of Duchenne muscular dystrophy (DMD) was noted very early on by both Meryon and Gowers (references in Chapter 2). In fact, as we have seen in Chapter 2, Gowers recognized that the disorder was limited to males and transmitted by healthy females, a mode of inheritance now recognized to be that of an X-linked recessive trait (Fig. 8.1).

Mode of inheritance

Evidence of X-linked recessive inheritance includes not only the typical pedigree pattern but also the fact that occasional female heterozygous carriers have had affected sons by different husbands. However, neither of these observations excludes the possibility that the disorder could be inherited as an autosomal dominant trait that is expressed only in males, so-called sex-limitation. Two lines of evidence refute this. First, the disorder has been recorded in females with XO Turner's syndrome, XO mosaicism, or with a structurally abnormal X chromosome or an XY chromosome constitution. Secondly, statistical evidence indicates that the proportion of cases due to new mutations more closely resembles that expected for an X-linked recessive trait than for an autosomal dominant trait with male limitation. However, until the 1980s, the disease locus did not appear to be within measurable distance of other known X-linked loci. However, using DNA probes as well as information generated by patients with

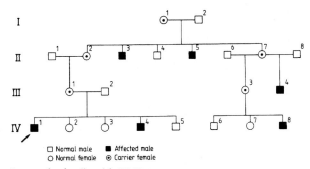

Fig. 8.1 Pedigree of a family with DMD.

cytogenetically identifiable deletions, the disease locus has now been shown to be located on the short arm of the X chromosome at position Xp2l.

Penetrance

Complex segregation analysis in a large number of families with the disease indicates that the gene for DMD is always fully penetrant.

Incidence

In order to determine the frequency of the responsible gene and its rate of mutation it is necessary to determine the population frequency of the disorder. This information is also essential in order to determine if various preventive measures are being effective, and to help in the planning of adequate resources and welfare services for affected families.

Incidence refers to the number of *new* cases occurring per unit of population. Prevalence, on the other hand, refers to *all cases present in the population*, either within a given period (so-called period prevalence rate) or at a particular point in time (so-called point prevalence rate) per unit of population at-risk at that time. In the case of DMD, prevalence, particularly after early childhood, would be less than the true incidence at birth because of increasing mortality.

Since the disorder is not clinically recognizable at birth, birth incidence is usually derived from knowing the number of normal boys born in the same years that affected boys were born. However, a small proportion of normal boys may die by the age at which affected boys are diagnosed. It has therefore been argued that incidence should perhaps be related not to the number of normal live births but rather to the number of normal children who survive to the age at which affected boys are diagnosed. But some affected boys may also die before clinical manifestations become evident. The best compromise seems to be to calculate incidence from the assumed frequency at birth as a proportion of all births.

Incidence may also be derived from prevalence by taking into account the probability of ascertaining affected individuals in the population and the probability of an individual developing the disease by a given age.

Some significant variations between the estimates of incidence and prevalence in various countries have been reported, including differences even within a single country such as the UK or Italy. The highest incidences between the 1960s and 1980s were reported in Emilia (north-east Italy, 390×10^{-6}), north-east England regions (311×10^{-6}), and the Erfurt region in Germany (307×10^{-6}), while the lowest incidences were recorded in Poland (140×10^{-6}) and

Table 8.1 DMD: prevalence in the population and incidence in live male births (LMB)*

Number affected	Total population	Prevalence (mean ± SE) × 10⁻⁶	Number affected	Total LMB	Incidence (mean ± SE) × 10⁻⁶
1956	46 282 453	42 ± 1	2 111	10 236 248	206 ± 4

* These data are based on some 50 reported studies covering the period 1939–1990.
(Detailed references can be found in the previous edition of this book.)

Friuli (Italy, 97×10^{-6}). Regarding population prevalence figures, in the same period of time they ranged upwards from 17.2×10^{-6} in Kumamoto (Japan) to 69.3×10^{-6} in Emilia (Italy). A summary of the incidence and prevalence data published from all over the world is given in Table 8.1.

Despite increasing awareness of the disease in recent years there has been no significant increase in reported incidences. It could be that any inflation by the inclusion of other forms of dystrophy in the past has been balanced in more recent studies by improved ascertainment of true cases. The overall incidence based on over 10 million live male births is $206 \pm 4 \times 10^{-6}$, or one case in 4 854. But this figure includes some seemingly abnormally low estimates. In several more recent and exhaustive studies birth incidence approaches 300×10^{-6} or roughly 1 in 3 500 male births (Emery 1991).

The birth incidence of the disease can also be determined by screening for a raised SCK level in the neonatal period (see Chapter 11, p. 173) and subsequently confirming the diagnosis by muscle histology followed by dystrophin studies and gene deletion analysis. These screening programmes first began in the 1970s with subsequent reports from New Zealand, Scotland, France, and Germany. Since then there have been a number of technological improvements and current results from several extensive studies are summarized in Table 8.2 where the overall incidence is given as $199 \pm 14 \times 10^{-6}$.

These studies clearly show that the neonatal screening for DMD is feasible and, coupled with molecular genetic testing and muscle biopsy, is effective in diagnosing affected children early. Currently, neonatal screening programmes are underway in several countries. There are, however, both practical and ethical issues that have so far prohibited a more widespread use of this early diagnostic technique. These will be discussed in detail in Chapter 11.

Changes in incidence in recent years

In recent years and perhaps more so in future, some reduction in the incidence of DMD might be expected as a result of several factors. Beginning in the 1950s there was an increase in interest in genetic counselling, and the

Table 8.2 Results of various neonatal screening programmes for DMD reported at the 14th ENMC Sponsored Workshop 'Screening for Muscular Dystrophy', 5–6 March 1992, Baarn, The Netherlands (Chairman: Professor G.-J. van Ommen).

Centre	Start of programme	Age tested	Total screened ($\times 10^3$)	False positive (%)	Proven DMD
Manitoba, Canada	1986	1–5 days	54	0.10	10
Lyons, France	1975	5 days 3 days	328	0.19 0.40	60
Philadelphia, USA	1986	1–4 days	49	0.30	10
Antwerp, Belgium	1975	5–7 days	150	0.02	25
Cardiff, Wales	1990	6–7 days	24	0.02	9
Germany*	1977	4 weeks–6 months	358	0.02	78
Total ($I = 199 \pm 14 \times 10^{-6}$)			963		192

* Voluntary screening.

mid-1960s saw the advent of carrier detection tests. Later, prenatal fetal sexing became possible so that a mother who was at high risk of having an affected son could request selective abortion of any male fetus in any subsequent pregnancy. Finally, in the recent past prenatal diagnosis of affected male fetuses has become possible using molecular genetic testing. Although this latter development is perhaps too recent to have had any major effect itself on incidence, genetic counselling and carrier detection studies in affected families might be predicted to have resulted in some reduction in incidence. In a well designed and careful study in western Japan a decrease in incidence from 223×10^{-6} for the period 1956–60 to 145×10^{-6} for the period 1976–80 was noted and attributed to the effects of genetic counselling (Takeshita *et al.* 1977; 1987).

Mutation rate

The rate at which the gene causing DMD mutates may be estimated either indirectly or directly.

Indirect estimation of mutation rate

For any X-linked recessive disorder if the reproductive fitness of affected individuals is f, and the incidence of the disease is I, then the mutation rate is

$$\text{Mutation rate} = \tfrac{1}{3} I (1 - f).$$

However, in DMD biological fitness is zero because affected boys do not procreate. Therefore the mutation rate is given by $\frac{1}{3}$.

If the incidence of the disorder is assumed to be around $200\text{–}300 \times 10^{-6}$, then the mutation rate is around $70\text{–}100 \times 10^{-6}$ genes per generation.

Direct estimation of mutation rate

In the direct method an attempt is made to estimate the actual number of new mutations among isolated cases. If a of b known female carriers have an abnormal SCK level, then the detection rate of carriers is a/b. If n isolated cases are born in a given period among N males born in the same period, and if c is the number of mothers of these n males who have an *abnormal* SCK level, then among these isolated cases (subject to sampling error) the number of *new* mutations will be

$$n - (bc/a)$$

and therefore the mutation rate is

$$(n - (bc/a))/N.$$

In one study (Gardner-Medwin 1970), 22 of 35 known carriers had raised SCK levels. Of 56 mothers of isolated cases, 15 had raised levels. Thus the proportion of new mutations (mothers are non-carriers) among isolated cases was

$$[56 - 15(35/22)]/56 = 0.574.$$

Over a 9-year period (1952–60), 43 isolated cases were born and therefore the number of new mutations was

$$(43)(0.574) = 24.682.$$

The total number of males born in this period who survived to age 5 (by which time almost all cases of DMD are diagnosed) was 236 200. Thus the mutation rate was

$$24.682/236\,200 = 105 \times 10^{-6}.$$

The estimates of the mutation rate by both these methods are considerably greater than values obtained for other X-linked disorders. For comparison some representative values for various genetic disorders are given in Table 8.3. The only disorder with a comparable mutation rate is neurofibromatosis but this is now known not to be a single genetic disease. The very high mutation rate in DMD is probably a reflection of the enormous size of the dystrophin gene, which therefore provides a bigger target for mutagenic agents.

Table 8.3 Average estimates of mutation rates for various genetic disorders (data from various sources)

Disorder	Mutation rate ($\times 10^{-6}$)
Autosomal dominants	
Achondroplasia	6–13
Retinoblastoma	5–12
Tuberous sclerosis	6–10.5
Polyposis coli	13
Neurofibromarosis	44–100
Huntington's chorea	5
Myotonic dystrophy	8–11
Autosomal recessives	
Albinism	28
Total colour blindness	28
Phenylketonuria	25
X-linked recessives	
Haemophilia A	32–57
Haemophilia B	2–3

Parental age and mutation rate

In X-linked recessive disorders possible effects of maternal or paternal age on mutation rates can be assessed separately by considering, respectively, maternal age in the case of mutant males, and the maternal grandfather's age in the case of mutant heterozygous mothers. The latter are mothers with no affected relatives other than sons (or who have only one affected son but a significantly elevated SCK level) where the new mutation can have occurred in the X-chromosome she inherited from her father.

None of the studies that have considered this problem have found any significant increase in the age of mothers of presumed new mutants. With regard to presumed mutant heterozygous mothers, the mean ages of both grandparents at the birth of these mothers can be compared with the mean ages of the mothers' spouses' parents at the birth of their spouse. In several studies the mean maternal grandfather's age was greater than the mean paternal grandfather's age (Table 8.4), but the differences were not statistically significant.

If there is any paternal age effect on the mutation rate in this disorder it would seem to be negligible. The results of these studies do not support the idea that the mutation rate in males is significantly different from that in females.

Table 8.4 Ages (years) of grandparents of cases of DMD where the mother is presumed to be a mutant heterozygote

Maternal grandparent			Paternal grandparent			Difference	Year of study
Number	Mean age	SD	Number	Mean age	SD		
Grandfathers							
26	34.3	6.14	22	30.9	6.42	+3.4	1977
15	35.1	7.03	15	31.4	6.43	+3.7	1980
82	34.1	7.33	81	33.9	7.56	+0.5	1982
Grandmothers							
26	30.5	4.87	24	27.8	5.47	+2.7	1977
14	30.4	6.63	16	27.4	5.48	+3.0	1980
82	30.3	7.06	82	29.0	6.07	+1.3	1982

Sex difference in mutation rate

It can be shown that, if a mother has an affected son but no one else in the family is affected, then the probability of her being a carrier is

$$(\mu + \nu)/(2\mu + \nu)$$

where μ is the mutation rate in female germ cells and ν is the mutation rate in male germ cells. The probability that she is *not* a carrier and that the son is therefore the result of a new mutation is

$$1 - [(\mu + \nu)/(2\mu + \nu)] = \mu/(2\mu + \nu),$$

which represents the proportion of new mutants, often designated as 'x'. If the mutation rates are the same in both males and females then x is one-third, if mutations occurred more frequently in the male then x approaches zero, and, if mutations occurred more frequently in the female, then x approaches one-half.

This is not just of academic importance because, if mutations were found to occur exclusively in the male, then all mothers with an affected son would be carriers, and this would be important in genetic counselling.

Several different methods have been devised for estimating x. Essentially there are three approaches:

- analysis of sibships;
- sex ratio of unaffected sibs;
- methods based on the results of carrier detection tests.

With regard to the sex ratio method, this is independent of ascertainment, and is based on the assumption that, among offspring of a *carrier*, affected boys, unaffected boys, and girls will, on average, occur in the ratio 1 : 1 : 2. Therefore the sex ratio (M : F) among unaffected sibs will be 1 : 2 (or 1 : 1.89 if corrected for the deviation of the sex ratio from 1). However, among the sibs of *new mutants* the sex ratio will be 1 : 1 (or 1 : 0.94 if corrected). The proportion of new mutants among isolated cases can be estimated by determining the sex ratio among the sibs of isolated cases.

Finally, with regard to carrier detection methods, these have usually been based on comparing the proportion of abnormal test results (the most reliable in the past being the SCK level) in known carriers with mothers of isolated cases. Thus, if i is the proportion of mothers of isolated cases with an elevated SCK level, d is the proportion of known carriers with an elevated SCK level, and P_i is the proportion of isolated cases among all cases assuming complete ascertainment in a given population, then

$$x = (1 - i/d)P_i.$$

The results of some 20 studies of the problem indicate that x would accumulate a value of 0.33, which assumes that mutations are equal in males and females.

The possibility of *germ-line mosaicism* must also be considered as a possible explanation for lower values of x. In an extensive study of a pooled sample of 1885 sibships from seven different countries, the proportion of sporadic cases was estimated to be 0.229 ± 0.026 (Barbujani *et al.* 1990). From these data it can be calculated that the upper 95 per cent confidence limit for x is 0.280 and therefore the proportion due to mosaicism in apparently non-carrier mothers would be expected to be at least 16 per cent. This figure is close to that obtained from molecular studies (see Chapter 11).

The increasing election by mothers, after the birth of an affected son, of family limitation and selective abortion in future pregnancies, may well invalidate the assumptions underlying these various approaches. These practices will lead to an increasing proportion of isolated cases and a decreasing sex ratio (M : F) in subsequent sibs.

Finally, a recent collaborative international investigation of the problem using DNA haplotypes in order to identify the origin of mutations within families indicates that the mutation rates in males and females are roughly equal (Muller *et al.* 1992).

So far it has been assumed that all cases result from a mutation in the germ cells. But if the male twins discordant for DMD reported by de Grouchy in 1963 were in fact identical, as the authors stated, then this raises the possibility that mutations may also occur after conception. Post-zygotic mutation would also account for a reported pair of monozygotic (MZ) twins being discordant for example for tuberous sclerosis. There could be other examples.

Summary and conclusions

Evidence from various sources, including pedigree studies, affected girls with X chromosome abnormalities, and statistical methods has shown that DMD is inherited as an X-linked recessive trait. The mutant gene is always fully penetrant and a subclinical, as opposed to a preclinical, form of the disease does not exist. Estimates of the incidence of the disorder, based on population surveys and neonatal screening, vary but are probably around $200-300 \times 10^{-6}$. This puts the mutation rate at around $70-100 \times 10^{-6}$ genes per generation, which is considerably greater than in any other disorder and reflects the enormous size of the dystrophin gene, which is therefore a greater target for mutagenic agents. A possible difference in mutation rates in male and female germ cells has been studied by considering maternal and grandpaternal age effects, as well as the proportion of isolated cases that could be due to new mutations. The results of all these investigations indicate that the mutation rates in male and female germ cells do not differ significantly and around one-third of isolated cases of the disease are due to new mutations.

References

Barbujani, G., Russo, A., Danieli, G.A., *et al.* (1990). Segregation analysis of 1885 DMD families: significant departure from the expected proportion of sporadic cases. *Human Genetics* **84**, 522–6.

Emery, A. (1991). Population frequencies of inherited neuromuscular diseases—a world survey. *Neuromuscular Disorders* **1**, 19–29.

Gardner-Medwin, D. (1970). Mutation rate in Duchenne type of muscular dystrophy. *Journal of Medical Genetics* **7**, 334–7.

Muller, B., Dechant, C., Meng, G., *et al.* (1992). Estimation of the male and female mutation rates in Duchenne muscular dystrophy (DMD). *Human Genetics* **89**, 204–6.

Takeshita, K., Yoshino, K., Kitahara, T., Nakashima, T., and Kaito, N. (1977). Survey of Duchenne type and congenital muscular dystrophy in Shimane, Japan. *Japanese Journal of Human Genetics* **22**, 43–7.

Takeshita, K., Kasagi, S., Mito, T., *et al.* (1987). Decreased incidence of Duchenne muscular dystrophy in Western Japan 1956–80. *Neuroepidemiology* **6**, 130–8.

Chapter 9

Molecular pathology

In order to unravel the molecular pathology of a disease where the basic biochemical defect is unknown, various approaches are possible. These have been well exemplified in the case of Duchenne muscular dystrophy (DMD). First, the gene has to be localized to a specific chromosome and then to a particular site on the chromosome. Secondly, armed with such information, DNA markers can be selected that are located in this particular region of the chromosome and, if they prove to be closely linked to the disease locus, they can be used for carrier detection and prenatal diagnosis. Thirdly, it may be possible, using molecular techniques, to 'walk the genome' from the DNA markers toward the mutant gene so as to eventually include the gene itself. As will be seen, however, there have been several other strategies pursued to isolate the Duchenne locus. Fourthly, having isolated the gene, or at least part of it, this can then be used as a 'gene-specific' probe for direct prenatal diagnosis and carrier detection. Finally, having isolated the gene, it is then possible by DNA amplification and sequencing to define the nature of the molecular defect and its product. Each of these steps will be described in relation to DMD, although much of the detail is really outside the scope of this book and is furnished in the relevant bibliography.

Localization of the Duchenne gene

An early clue as to the specific location of the Duchenne locus came from the study of rare cases of a Duchenne-like disorder in girls with X/autosome translocations (Ray et al. 1985). The first cases were described in the late 1970s. Since then some 20 or so similar cases have been reported. Full details with references are given in the 2nd edition of this book. In each case the findings have been consistent with the diagnosis of a muscular dystrophy with grossly elevated serum creatine kinase (SCK) levels and myopathic changes on electromyography (EMG) and muscle pathology. Most have been clinically similar to DMD, although in some cases the disorder seemed less severe and perhaps more like Becker muscular dystrophy (BMD). Some girls have been mentally retarded. All, however, have had a reciprocal translocation between an autosome and the X chromosome and, since these are balanced translocations with

Table 9.1 Expression of X-linked disorders in females with various X/autosome translocations

Disorder	X breakpoint
DMD and BMD	Xp21
Anhidrotic ectodermal dysplasia	Xq12
Aicardi's syndrome	Xp22
Hunter's syndrome	Xq28
Aarskog syndrome	Xq13
Incontinentia pigmenti	Xp11
Lowe's syndrome	Xq25
Menkes syndrome	Xq13

no apparent loss of chromosomal material, these girls might have been expected to be normal. In such X/autosome translocations, however, it is the normal X that tends to be preferentially inactivated, with the result that genes on the derived (der) X are expressed. It could therefore be that the mothers of these girls were heterozygous carriers and that the maternal X chromosome carrying the mutant gene was involved in the translocation. However, this is unlikely because in only two instances has there been any suggestion that the mother might be a carrier and that the translocation chromosome was, in fact, of paternal origin Also, the parents of these girls have had normal chromosomes and we are therefore left to conclude that both the translocation as well as the disease must have arisen *de novo* in the affected girls.

Since different autosomes were involved in the various translocations but the breakpoint on the X chromosome was *always* in the region of Xp21, the most likely explanation is that the translocation in some way disrupted the normal gene at Xp21, which then resulted in the disease. The mutant gene was therefore presumed to be located at this point on the X chromosome (Fig. 9.1). There is considerable variation in clinical severity among girls with X/autosome translocations and a Duchenne-like disorder. It seems possible that the phenotype may well depend on the proportion of cells in which the der X is active. The milder the phenotype, the lower the proportion of cells in which the active X chromosome is the der X, and therefore the greater the proportion of cells in which the active X chromosome is the normal X. In fact, the published data indicate that the proportion of cells in which the active X is the der X was somewhat lower in cases considered to be mild.

X/autosome translocations involving other breakpoints on the X chromosome have also been described. In these cases as well, the expression of various

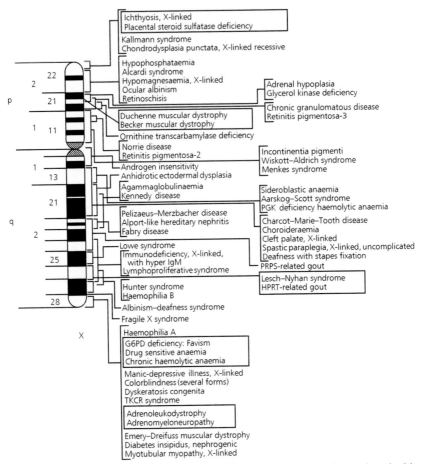

Fig. 9.1 Gene map of the X-chromosome and its banding pattern. (Reproduced with permission from McKusick (1992, p. cci).)

X-linked disorders could be attributed to the disruption of the normal alleles at the respective loci (Table 9.1).

While studies of X/autosome translocations in females with muscular dystrophy were in progress, a unique case was described that further confirmed the location of the Duchenne locus. This concerned a boy with DMD and some degree of mental retardation, who also exhibited chronic granulomatous disease, McLeod syndrome (reduced antigenicity of the red cell Kell blood group), and a form of retinitis pigmentosa. High-resolution chromosome banding studies revealed that the band Xp21 appeared to be slightly reduced in size, and molecular studies confirmed that the affected boy had a small interstitial deletion in this region. This deletion presumably removed DNA sequences at the DMD locus as well as at other adjacent loci thus producing the clinical phenotypes. This case further supported the idea that the Duchenne locus was at Xp21. It also indicated that the loci for these different disorders are clustered together. In fact, various associations of these different disorders have been reported in males: chronic granulomatous disease with McLeod syndrome; McLeod syndrome with raised SCK levels and a subclinical myopathy; chronic granulomatous disease with McLeod syndrome and raised SCK levels; chronic granulomatous disease with DMD; chronic granulomatous disease, McLeod syndrome, DMD, and a form of retinitis pigmentosa. The gene for ornithine transcarbamylase (OTC) is also localized to Xp21 and has been shown to be relatively closely linked to the Duchenne locus. A small but visible deletion associated with OTC and glycerol kinase deficiencies and X-linked adrenal hypoplasia has been described. Also, a deletion in the same region of the X chromosome has been found in boys with a myopathy, glycerol kinase deficiency, and adrenal insufficiency. This triad has also been reported when there is no visible deletion, but a deletion may then be detected using an appropriate DNA probe. The triad may also be associated with other abnormalities. Glycerol kinase deficiency and adrenal hypoplasia have been recorded in different male members of a particular family but in the absence of a myopathy, and the glycerol kinase locus is clearly distinct from the Duchenne locus. Åland Island eye disease can also occur in association with DMD, glycerol kinase deficiency, and congenital adrenal hypoplasia. We know of another instance with a large deletion in three siblings with BMD, glycerol kinase deficiency, adrenal hypoplasia, undescended testes, and mental retardation, which led to the identification of a novel gene (interleukin-1 receptor related protein, IL1RAPL1). Interestingly, in these brothers the dystrophin gene was fused tail-to-tail with the *IL1RAPL1* gene. Mutations in this gene have been also reported in non-specific X-linked mental retardation.

On the basis of these reports of overlapping phenotypes it is possible to order the responsible gene loci (Fig. 9.2). Because of the involvement of contiguous genes, these have been referred to as contiguous gene syndromes. This arrangement of the disease gene loci around the Duchenne locus has now been confirmed by detailed gene mapping studies.

Cases of DMD with no other associated abnormalities but with a microscopically evident interstitial deletion at Xp21 are very much the exception. Such cases have been described by several authors, where the deletion was large enough to be visible but was presumably not sufficiently extensive to include any adjacent gene loci. In the vast majority of cases of DMD, however, no deletion or any other alteration is microscopically evident in the region of

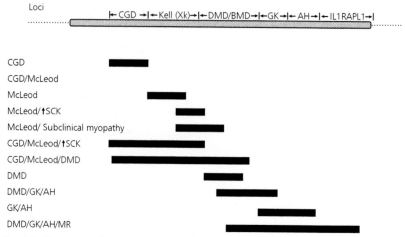

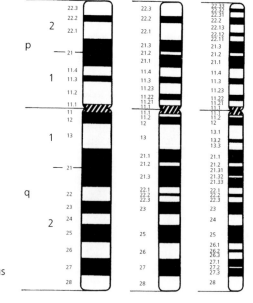

Fig. 9.2 Diagrammatic representation of contiguous gene syndromes involving chronic granulomatous disease (CGD), McLeod syndrome (Kell), DMD, BMD, glycerol kinase deficiency (GK), adrenal hypoplasia (AH), and mental retardation secondary to mutations in the interleukin receptor 1-like gene (IL1RALP1).

Fig. 9.3 Diagrammatic representation of the high-resolution banding patterns that can be delineated on the X chromosome by various techniques.

Xp21 even with high-resolution banding. Such techniques reveal that the band Xp21 can be subdivided into three regions (Fig. 9.3) and, when applied to lymphoblastoid cell lines from females with a Duchenne-like disorder and an X/autosome translocation, the breakpoint has been found to be in subband

Xp212 or in Xp211. It can be calculated that the DNA represented in the sub-bands Xp211, Xp212, and Xp213 is around 5 000, 2 000, and 4 000 kilobases (kb), respectively (1 kb = 1 000 base pairs of DNA). From these cytogenetic studies the chromosomal region involved in some way with DMD/BMD would therefore span more than 1 000 kb of DNA. In fact, these results have been confirmed by later genomic studies that have shown that the dystrophin locus spans approximately 3 megabases (mb), constituting roughly 3 per cent of chromosome X.

Linked DNA markers

Between genes there are large stretches of DNA, the functions of which are still largely unknown. Within this DNA are variations in nucleotide sequences or single nucleotide variations that have no apparent phenotypic effects on the host organism and are inherited in a Mendelian fashion. These changes in base sequence, which occur about once in every 100 base pairs, can be identified because they can alter the DNA site normally cleaved by a particular restriction enzyme since these enzymes cleave DNA at sequence-specific sites. Thus, a change in base sequence in a segment of DNA will, with a particular restriction enzyme, result in different-sized fragments in different individuals. These genotypic changes can be recognized in different ways. Until the early 1990s they could only be studied by the different mobilities of the restriction fragments on gel electrophoresis. The fragments were identified by using an appropriate 'probe', a labelled DNA fragment that will hybridize with, and thereby detect, complementary sequences among the DNA fragments produced by a restriction enzyme (Southern blot). These variations in nucleotide sequences are referred to as restriction fragment length polymorphisms (RFLPs). Their interest lies in the fact that the demonstration of linkage between an RFLP and the locus for a particular genetic disease can be useful for carrier detection and prenatal diagnosis. Also, if the chromosomal site of an RFLP were already known, it could furnish information on the site of a disease locus to which it proved to be closely linked.

More recently, the discovery of polymorphic microsatellite markers and of single nucleotide polymorphisms (SNPs) has greatly enhanced the possibility of detecting variations between individuals. The former typically are represented by stretches of di- or trinucleotides that are often highly polymorphic in the general population. They represent an advantage compared to RFLP because they can be easily assessed following a simple polymerase chain reaction (PCR) assay, they often have a significantly higher heterozygosity index, and are randomly located in the genome at intervals that, on average, are less than 1 map unit or centimorgan (cM; 1 cM is roughly equal to 1 000 kb or 106 base pairs (bp)) apart. This means that the majority of genes will have several polymorphic microsatellite markers located in close proximity, or within the introns of the genes themselves. This is the case also of the dystrophin gene, in which a number of intragenic polymorphic microsatellite markers have been identified and are listed in Appendix G. They therefore represent very powerful tools for studying linkage of a particular locus in family studies.

A hypothetical example of the co-inheritance of an RFLP and an X-linked recessive disorder is given in Fig. 9.4. Here it is assumed there is a polymorphism at restriction site B—the absence of the site is called allele-1 and the presence of the site is allele-2. When the restriction enzyme cuts the DNA in one chromosome at sites A and C it generates a single fragment of size 10 kb, which corresponds to allele-1. If the enzyme cuts the DNA not only at sites A and C but also at B, two fragments will now be generated of sizes 7 and 3 kb, respectively, which correspond to allele-2. Polymorphic genotypes can therefore be deduced from the pattern of bands on an electrophoretic gel. In this example, grandmother (I_2) and mother (II_2) are both heterozygous for the RFLP and both carry the X-linked recessive disorder. Since both affected males have allele-2 it would appear that allele-2 and the disorder are co-inherited in this family. That is, they are both on the same X chromosome.

By studying individuals in a family in which an RFLP and an X-linked recessive disorder are inherited it is possible to estimate how frequently crossing-over occurs between them. Thus, in this example, if the unaffected son III_1 had also inherited allele-2, there would appear to have been at least one cross-over (or recombinant) out of four meioses. By studying a number of informative

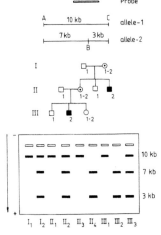

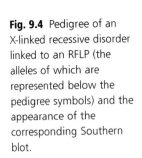

Fig. 9.4 Pedigree of an X-linked recessive disorder linked to an RFLP (the alleles of which are represented below the pedigree symbols) and the appearance of the corresponding Southern blot.

families in this way, the frequency of recombination can be determined. Recombination frequency, usually designated as θ, is related to the distance between the gene loci concerned—1 per cent recombination being equivalent to a distance of 1 cM. When loci are some distance apart then the error rate in diagnosis will be equal to θ at each meiosis.

With regard to linkage with DMD, the first step was to isolate a relevant DNA sequence. In 1981, Davies and her colleagues isolated the first DNA sequences from cloned fragments derived from the human X chromosome, the so-called X genomic library. The location of these cloned sequences was then determined by various methods. These included studying somatic cell hybrids with a full complement of Chinese hamster or mouse chromosomes and different extents of the human X chromosome. Another method of localizing a DNA sequence was by *in situ* hybridization whereby the sequence was labelled and hybridized directly to a metaphase chromosome preparation. One of the cloned sequences, designated RC8, turned out to be located on the short arm of X chromosome. Using this as a probe, it detected a polymorphism with the restriction enzyme Taq I, and by studying several families the polymorphism detected by RC8 (now called DXS9) proved to be linked to DMD. Shortly afterwards, a different probe (L1 .28) detected another polymorphism (DXS7) on the opposite side of Xp21, and it was found that the Duchenne locus lay between the two. Both markers eventually turned out to be about 15 cM on either side (referred to as 'flanking' or 'bridging') the Duchenne locus. Not only was this a landmark in the history of the disease but it was the first disorder shown to be linked to an RFLP (Davies *et al.* 1983).

Around the same time, others showed that BMD was linked to DXS7 (L1.28). Subsequently, it was also shown to be linked to DXS9 (RC8) and to other DNA markers at roughly similar genetic distances to those in DMD. These findings therefore indicated that DMD and BMD could either be allelic or that the two loci could be very close together in the same region of the X chromosome. We now know that they are, in fact, allelic. Interestingly, Emery–Dreifuss muscular dystrophy was shown to be linked to colour blindness and to DNA markers located at Xq28, which indicated that the responsible gene mutation was not allelic with DMD and BMD. We now know that the gene responsible for X-linked Emery–Dreifuss muscular dystrophy is the *STA* gene, located at Xq28.

The identification of dystrophin intragenic polymorphic microsatellite markers has recently improved the study of carriers in families with DMD or BMD. A complete list of the various dystrophin gene polymorphisms can be found in Appendix G.

Isolation of the Duchenne gene

The most obvious approach to eventually isolating the Duchenne gene itself would *a priori* have been to 'walk the genome' from a closely linked probe toward the gene, so as to eventually include it. This could be done by studying overlapping clones of DNA sequences. There are several reasons, however, why this approach proved difficult. Even a very closely linked marker only 1 cM from the disease locus is a million base pairs away, and it would be extremely difficult to know if one were moving closer or further away by this strategy. Other methods seemed more likely to succeed.

One approach, pursued by Worton and his colleagues in Toronto, Canada, was to isolate the junctional region in an X/autosome translocation associated with a Duchenne-like disorder in a female. They chose a translocation involving chromosome 21, which they showed split the block of genes encoding ribosomal RNA on the short arm of chromosome 21 (Worton *et al.* 1984). They then used ribosomal DNA probes to identify the junctional fragment in clones derived from the region of the translocation site. The region spanning the translocation breakpoint, and which presumably contained at least part of the Duchenne locus, was then cloned. A sequence derived from the clone was found to detect an RFLP that was very closely linked to DMD. This probe (referred to as XJ probe) failed to hybridize with DNA from the occasional patient with DMD, indicating that in these boys there is a deletion of the region complementary to the probe.

Kunkel and colleagues in Boston approached the problem in a different and particularly ingenious way. They extracted DNA from a patient with a large deletion spanning the locus. The DNA was then sheared by sonication which produces DNA fragments with irregular ends. DNA from a 49, XXXXY lymphoid cell line was cleaved with the restriction enzyme *Mbo*I. The two sets of fragments were then mixed and heated in order to disassociate the DNA strands. These were then allowed to reassociate in the presence of phenol (so-called phenol-enhanced reassociation technique, PERT). Under appropriate conditions, and with the patient's DNA in excess, most of the reassociated molecules will have sheared ends and a few will be hybrid molecules with one sheared end and one *Mbo*I 'sticky end'. However, those sequences in the control not represented in the patient's DNA (where they are deleted) will *not* hybridize with the patient's DNA. Perforce, they will only hybridize between themselves and therefore consist of perfectly reassociated molecules with two *Mbo*I ends. Only the last can be ligated into an appropriately cleaved plasmid and be cloned (Kunkel *et al.* 1985). In this way a library of cloned sequences (referred to as PERT probes), corresponding to the portion of DNA deleted in the affected boy, was produced. These have detected several RFLPs closely linked to the Duchenne locus and, like Worton's probes, they also detected small deletions in a proportion of affected boys (Monaco *et al.* 1985) which are of different lengths in different families (Kunkel *et al.* 1986).

It should be noted that the probes isolated by Worton (XJ) and Kunkel (PERT) have shown recombination with DMD ($\theta \cong 0.05$) thus further indicating that the Duchenne locus is very large. In fact, recombination between markers at the two extremes of the locus is at least 10 per cent. But recombination may not be uniform throughout the locus. A hotspot, for example, is centred around DXS 164 (PERT 87).

Deletions

The Xp21 locus has been cloned and, using cDNA probes derived in this way, approximately 70 per cent of cases of DMD and over 80 per cent of cases of BMD have been found to have gene deletions. These findings have two important implications. First, if the deletion involves a significant part of the gene, then it might be expected that the affected individual could mount an immune response if exposed to the missing gene product and this could make replacement therapy difficult. Secondly, it is possible to track down the origin of the deletions, and identify the occurrence of *de novo* events. This is illustrated in Fig. 9.5 based on two families. Using a particular probe (PERT 87–8) an RFLP was detected with the enzyme *Bst*XI reflected in two DNA fragments of sizes 4.4 and 2.2 kb (say, allele-1 and allele-2, respectively).

- In family A, grandmother (I_2) is either homozygous for allele-2 or hemizygous because one allele has been deleted. Her daughter (II_1) has no allele-2 which she should have inherited from her mother. She is therefore heterozygous for the deletion that is evident in her affected son (III_1) who is therefore *not* a new mutation.

- In family B both grandmother and mother are heterozygous for the RFLP and neither allele is deleted. However, one of the alleles is deleted in the affected son who must therefore be a *new* mutation.

Though up to 70 per cent of cases of DMD have a deletion, a proportion have a gene duplication, which probably results from unequal sister-chromatid exchange. The rate of duplication might have been underestimated in the past and, in fact, up to 15 per cent of DMD might result from this mechanism (Abbs *et al.*, personal observation).

Regarding the methods for detecting deletions and duplications, most diagnostic laboratories currently use a system of multiplex PCRs, in which several exons are co-amplified in the same reaction tube (Chapter 4). Since the deletions and duplication almost invariably involve two regions of the gene (the

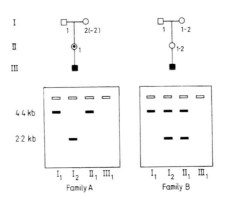

Fig. 9.5 Two families in which affected boys have a gene deletion. The alleles of an informative RFLP are represented below the pedigree symbols and the appearances of the corresponding Southern blots are shown.

5′ and the 3′ deletion 'hot spots'), not all 79 exons need to be analysed for identifying mutations. In practice, by studying only 19 exons in two multiplex PCR assayes, approximately 98 per cent of deletions can be identified. This test is considerably cheaper than the Southern blot and has the advantage that it can be run in hours. In addition, it can be relatively easily used under quantitative conditions, therefore allowing the dosage of amplified DNA to be established, an important point in carrier studies and in duplication detection. The disadvantage of the multiplex PCR assay occurs when the deletions endpoint fall outside the region covered by the 19 exons studied. In these cases the determination of the effect of the deletion/duplication on the reading frame is impossible.

The remaining cases are secondary to point mutations, microdeletions, and intronic rearrangements and splice site mutations. Several methods have been used to look at point mutations and other small gene rearrangements, and will be discussed later.

Origin of deletions

The precise mechanism responsible for deletions is not known. However, the effect of enviromental mutagenic agents might well play a role in this as has been demonstrated in animal models. The occurrence of deletion hot spots is intriguing as it suggests that the size of the gene is not the only factor involved. The role of repetitive elements (Line; Alu sequences) has been recently implicated in specific rearrangements (Suminaga et al. 2000). For example, the sequencing of the breakpoint in patients with deletions of exons 2–7 has identified the presence of an Alu sequence in intron 1, 25 kb downstream from the 3′ end of exon 1 that was joined directly to an Line1 sequence in intron 7, 4.5kb downstream from the 3′ end of exon 7. This novel recombination event therefore joined non-homologous Alu and L1 repeats. Furthermore, the nucleotide sequence of a deletion junction fragment from a DMD patient with a deletion of exon 44 showed that the proximal breakpoint of the deletion in intron 43 fell within the sequence of a transposon-like element normally present in a complete form in intron 43 of the dystrophin gene (Pizzuti *et al.* 1992). Considering the frequent occurrence of repetitive elements in the introns of the dystrophin gene, it is likely that they play a role in the origin of deletions. Furthermore, the bimodal distribution of deletions within the dystrophin gene (Fig. 4.13, p. 66) coincided with the bimodal distributions of recombination hot spots. Possibly the latter also therefore contributes to the origin of some deletions, as a result of possible breakage–fusion.

The dystrophin gene

The dystrophin gene was isolated and characterized by first using PERT and XJ probes to identify relevant mRNA transcripts in human skeletal muscle. The corresponding cDNA was then cloned and sequenced. The gene proved to be some 3 000 kb in length, now known to consist of at least 86 exons (including at least 7 promoters) of mean size 0.2 kb and introns of mean size 35 kb. The gene is transcribed into a 14 kb mRNA. Thus, the actual coding sequences represent less than 1 per cent of the nucleotide composition of the gene locus.

Muscle dystrophin is not the only product of the Duchenne gene locus. There are three full-length isoforms that have the same number of exons as the main muscle (M) isoform but derived from different promoters (B isoform, where B stands for brain, and P isoform, for cerebellar Purkinje neurons).

Multiple truncated isoforms also exist, generated from promoters located within the dystrophin gene. These are indicated by their molecular weight and named DP280; Dp140; DP116, and Dp71, generated by promoters located in introns 30, 45, 56, and 63, respectively. Several of these isoforms are relevant for the function of dystrophin in brain and have been described in detail in Chapter 6.

Dystrophin

Using polyclonal antibodies directed against fusion proteins produced in bacteria from cDNA, the protein product of the Xp21 locus has been identified (Hoffman *et al.* 1987). It has been named *dystrophin* and, as would be predicted, is a very large protein (Fig. 9.6).

The main isoform expressed in muscle has a molecular weight of 427 kDa consisting of 3 685 amino acids. It is a rod-shaped protein composed of four domains:

- *N*-terminal domain with homology to α-actinin and composed of 240 amino acids;

427 kD with 4 domains of 3685 aa

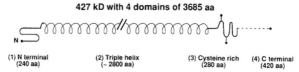

| (1) N terminal | (2) Triple helix | (3) Cysteine rich | (4) C terminal |
| (240 aa) | (~ 2800 aa) | (280 aa) | (420 aa) |

Fig. 9.6 The dystrophin molecule. aa, Amino acids.

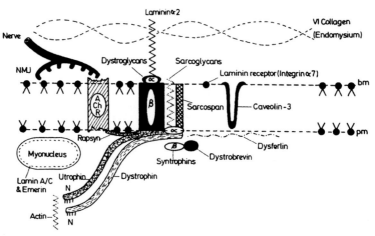

Fig. 9.7 Schematic representation of the various proteins involved directly or indirectly in different forms of muscular dystrophy. The precise relationships of these various proteins is not yet entirely clear. bm, Basement membrane (basl lamina); pm, plasma membrane (plasmalemma); NMJ, neuromuscular junction; AChR, acetyl choline receptor. (Taken with permission from Emery (2000).)

- central rod domain formed by a succession of 25 triple helical repeats similar to spectrin, and composed of roughly 3 000 amino acids;
- cysteine-rich domain composed of 280 amino acids;
- C-terminal domain composed of 420 amino acids.

That dystrophin shares many features with spectrin and α-actinin indicates that it too is a cytoskeletal protein. Early on it was shown to be localized to muscle cell membranes. It is a costameric protein forming a lattice that encircles the muscle fibre and attaches the sarcomeres to the sarcolemma. Dystrophin is not directly inserted into the membrane but is inserted via β-dystroglycan, a glycoprotein that is part of the dystrophin–glycoprotein complex (Fig. 9.7). The role of this complex in the pathogenesis of muscular dystrophy will be discussed in Chapter 10.

But, as we have seen, dystrophin is not a single protein but exists as a number of isoforms. Regarding the shorter isoforms, they all differ at their N-terminus, while they share with the full-length isoform the cysteine-rich domain and C-terminus. These shorter isoforms all lack therefore the actin-binding domain, while they share the dystroglycan-, dystrobrevin-, and syntrophin-binding domains, suggesting that they are capable of interaction with similar proteins at their C-terminus (Fig 10.1).

The presence of so many different isoforms and of dystrophin on different specialized membrane surfaces implies multiple functional roles for dystrophin proteins. The nature of these roles is as yet not fully understood, but is probably relevant in the distribution and extent of involvement of different tissues in DMD and BMD as a consequence of mutations at the Xp21 locus.

Molecular pathology and phenotype

There is no simple relationship between the extent of a mutation and the resultant clinical disease. For example, the deletions of small exons such as exon 44 or a comparatively minute deletion of 52 bp out of 88 bp in exon 19 result in classical DMD. On the other hand, large deletions involving nearly 50 per cent of the gene have been described in patients with BMD. Similarly, a massive duplication of more than 400 000 bp within the central region of the gene resulted in a dystrophin of approximately 600 kDa, but yet the patient only had a mild BMD. The effects on the phenotype depend, therefore, not so much on the extent of a deletion/duplication but on whether or not it disrupts the reading frame.

Frame-shift hypothesis

The milder BMD results from mutations that maintain the reading frame (in-frame), resulting in an abnormal but partially functional dystrophin, but in DMD mutations disrupt the reading frame (frame-shift) so that virtually no dystrophin is produced (Fig. 9.8). This reading frame hypothesis (Monaco *et al.* 1988) holds for over 90 per cent of cases. But exceptions do occur such as mild BMD with a frame-shift deletion or DMD with in-frame deletions. It is important to be aware of these cases as they might lead to diagnostic confusion.

Regarding cases of BMD with a frame-shift deletion, these involve deletions or duplications in the 5' end of the gene (exons 3–7; 5–7; 3–6) but also exons 51, 49–50, 47–52, 44, or 45. Moreover, rare patients with BMD despite truncation mutations (such as single nucleotide changes leading to a non-sense mutation) have also been described. These patients succeed in producing dystrophin by using exon skipping via alternative splicing (see Chapter 13) or in-frame translational re-initiation. Finally, splice site mutations predicted to lead to a out-of-frame deletion but actually resulting in larger deletions leading to restoration of the open reading frame (ORF) have also been described in BMD.

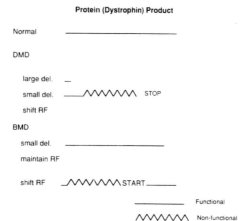

Fig. 9.8 Simplified diagram of the effects of mutations in the dystrophin gene on the gene product that maintain or disrupt (shift) the reading frame (RF).

On the whole, dystrophin amounts on muscle histochemistry or Western blot analysis correlate better with the phenotype than 'genetic prediction' especially in BMD, and various studies have reported figures in excess of 10 per cent for exceptions to the reading frame rule. Most investigators now believe that the hypothetical effect of a deletion on the ORF of dystrophin needs to be confirmed on muscle histochemistry in order to avoid a misdiagnosis. These patients are able to produce dystrophin that, though reduced in quantity and in molecular weight in case of deletions, or increased in molecular weight in case of duplications, retains partial function.

There is, however, some controversy as to whether the dystrophin level helps in predicting the severity of BMD. Some authors have commented on the lack of a simple correlation between dystrophin quantity and phenotype once all BMD patients are analysed together. On the other hand, when BMD patients with identical deletions in the 3′ hot spots are grouped together, the severity of the phenotype broadly correlates with the amount of dystrophin produced.

In an extensive study of patients with DMD with frame-shift mutations, the size of muscle dystrophin, detected at greatly reduced levels, agreed closely with that expected if the reading frame were restored and translation proceeded. Even the very low levels of muscle dystrophin in DMD may therefore have some functional significance. There is a correlation between the amount of dystrophin in these cases and the severity of the disease as assessed by the age at becoming confined to a wheelchair, although it is not clear how much of the phenotypic variability observed in DMD could be attributed in this way.

Exceptions to the reading frame rule occur not only in BMD but also in DMD. It is worth mentioning them as they may cause diagnostic confusion.

These patients typically have in-frame deletions that are nevertheless associated with a severe phenotype. In particular, most of these patients have relatively large deletions in the 5′ region extending into the mid-rod domain, for example, deletions removing exons 3–31 and 3–25, 4–41, 4–18, and 3–13. These deletions involve the 5′ principal putative actin-binding site of dystrophin and they are therefore likely to directly affect the interaction of dystrophin and actin, or affect it indirectly following an abnormal folding of dystrophin (Norwood *et al.* 2000).

Mutation site

Although deletions (and occasional duplications) can occur almost anywhere in the dystrophin gene, most occur in two 'hot-spots'. These have been referred to as the central high-frequency deletion region (HFDR) and the proximal HFDR (Fig. 4.12). The central HFDR is located approximately 1 200 kb from the 5′ end of the gene, clustered around exons 45–55. The proximal HFDR is located approximately 500 kb from the 5′ end of the gene, clustered around the first 20 exons. The clusters of these two hot spots represent the basis for using the multiplex PCR technique, which, by screening only 19 of the dystrophin exons, identifies approximately 98 per cent of all deletions.

Various authors have shown that proximal (5′) deletions are more common in familial cases and distal deletions in isolated cases. A 'proximal' new mutant has a greater risk of recurrence, of about 30 per cent, and a 'distal' new mutant has a lesser risk of recurrence of about 4 per cent.

The majority of out-of-frame (frame-shift) deletions in these regions, as well as elsewhere, result in severe DMD. Most of these cases have virtually no dystrophin. A few missense mutations with residual expression of dystrophin have been described in patients with DMD. The most convincing of these was reported in exon 69, in the β-dystroglycan binding site. This patient followed a severe DMD course despite the residual production of dystrophin, further reinforcing the importance of the interaction between β-dystroglycan and dystrophin for the function of the complex (Lenk *et al.* 1996)

A most interesting finding is that in-frame deletions of the central region of the gene that remove almost 50 per cent of the dystrophin can result in a mild phenotype. The resultant significantly truncated dystrophin is therefore adequate for almost normal muscle function. Furthermore, some deletions within this region may produce myalgia and muscle cramps but no weakness, or even no symptoms at all or merely a raised SCK level. We have studied three multigeneration families in whom an in-frame deletion of the central rod domain of the dystrophin gene, involving either exons 32–44 or 48–51 or 48–53, was only associated with elevation of SCK.

Rare and unusual dystrophin gene mutations have also been associated with X-linked dilated cardiomyopathy. This condition is a disease of heart muscle in which skeletal muscle is clinically not affected, although slight elevation of SCK has been documented in several affected families. Affected males develop symptoms of cardiac failure in the second or third decade of life. Cardiac transplant may be the only therapy possible in some severely affected males. We now know that this condition, initially mapped to the same locus as DMD and BMD, is a rare allelic variant of these two disorders. Most of the reported mutations occur in the 5′ of the gene (see Table 9.2) and selectively affect the expression of dystrophin in the heart. Detailed characterization of these cases may eventually clarify the differences in dystrophin transcriptional pathways between skeletal and cardiac muscle (for a review see Ferlini *et al.* 1999).

Table 9.2 Mutations of the dystrophin gene in X-linked dilated cardiomyopathy

Dystrophin gene mutation	Age of patients at study or death	Prognosis	CK
Muscle exon/intron 1 junction deletion	13	Death	High
Muscle exon 1 3′ splice site point mutation	24	Death*	Normal
Muscle exon 1 3′ splice site point mutation	11	Death	High
Splicing point mutation in intron 1 of muscle transcript	12	Death	High
Insertion of L1 element in muscle exon 1	17	Death	High
Insertion of L1 element in muscle exon 1	10	Death	High
Exons 45–48 deletion	39	Alive	Normal
Exons 45–55 deletion	36	Alive	High
Exon 48 deletion	17	Alive	High
Exon 48 deletion	24	Alive*	Normal
Exons 48–49 deletion	24	Alive	High
Exons 48–51 deletion	30	Alive	High
Exons 48–53 deletion	50	Alive	Normal
Exons 49–51 deletion	50	Death*	Normal
Exons 2–7 duplication	20	Alive*	High
Exon 9 point mutation	21	Death	High
Intron 11 deletion	16	Death*	High
Exon 29 point mutation	21	Death*	High
Exon 35 missense mutation	12	Death	High

* heart transplantation

These data indicate that there is a wide spectrum of abnormalities associated with mutations at the Xp21 locus. In fact, there may be healthy males in the population who have small defects in the central rod region of the dystrophin protein that may only be expressed under stress, such as muscle cramps after exercise or excessive muscle fatigue in later life. We are starting to understand the relationship between the effects of different mutations within the Xp21 locus and cardiac function. For example, a mutation that does not cause weakness might conceivably affect cardiac muscle in some way in later life in an otherwise healthy individual. We demonstrated this in two cases of X-linked dilated cardiomyopathy with 'typical BMD deletions', involving exons 48–49 in one case and exons 49–51 in the other. Intriguingly, SCK levels were entirely normal in this latter case.

Summary and conclusion

Several females with DMD and X/autosome translocations have been described, the breakpoint on the X chromosome always being at Xp21. This, and the fact that a unique case of DMD was found with a microscopically visible deletion in this same region of the X chromosomes, pointed to the disease locus being located at this point. Several RFLPs, which are polymorphisms due to the presence or absence of a particular restriction site, and, more recently, microsatellite polymorphic markers and SNPs have been identified around Xp21 and linked to the Duchenne locus. Information on linked markers can be used for prenatal diagnosis and, in conjunction with SCK levels, can be used in carrier detection in families without a deletion. Intragenic markers are now also available where the possibility of errors due to recombination are significantly reduced.

The analysis of the dystrophin gene by either Southern blot or multiplex PCR is able to identify submicroscopic gene deletions in up to 70 per cent of cases of DMD and BMD and duplications in 10–15 per cent of cases. The remaining cases carry point mutations that are spread throughout the entire gene making their detection technically difficult.

Finally, the Duchenne gene has been cloned and studied and has proved to be at least 3 000 kb in length and to consist of at least 86 exons. The gene product has been identified and called dystrophin. This is a very large protein, which is present in only very small amounts in normal muscle. It is virtually absent or nonfunctional in muscle in patients with DMD and truncated, presumably semifunctional, in BMD. It is associated with muscle cell membranes via glycoprotein forming a dystrophin–glycoprotein complex. Disruption of this complex, consequent on a deficiency of dystrophin, initiates the train of events that ultimately leads to muscle cell death. Dystrophin exists in a number of different isoforms (dystrophin-related proteins) with different tissue distributions. The effects of mutations at the Xp21 locus on these dystrophin isoforms might well explain the distribution and extent of involvement of different tissues in DMD.

References

Davies, K.E., Pearson, P.L., Harper, P.S., *et al.* (1983). Linkage analysis of two cloned DNA sequences flanking the Duchenne muscular dystrophy locus on the short arm of the human X chromosome. *Nucleic Acids Research* **11**, 2303–12.

Emery, A.E.H. (2000). Emery-Dreifuss muscular dystrophy – a 40-year retrospective. *Neuromuscular Disorders* **10**, 228–32.

Emery, A.E.H. (ed.) (2001). *The muscular dystrophies.* Oxford University Press, Oxford.

Ferlini, A., Sewry, C.A., Melis, M.A., Mateddu, A., and Muntoni, F. (1999). X-linked dilated cardiomyopathy and the dystrophin gene. *Neuromuscular Disorders* **9**, 339–46.

Hoffman, E.P., Brown, R.H., and Kunkel, L.M. (1987). Dystrophin: the protein product of the Duchenne muscular dystrophy locus. *Cell* **51**, 915–28.

Kunkel, L.M., Monaco, A.P., Middlesworth, W., Ochs, H.D., and Latt, S.A. (1985). Specific cloning of DNA fragments absent from the DNA of a male patient with an X chromosome deletion. *Proceedings of the National Academy of Sciences, USA* **82**, 4778–82.

Kunkel, L.M., Hejtmancik, J.F., Caskey, C.T., *et al.* (1986). Analysis of deletions in DNA from patients with Becker and Duchenne muscular dystrophy. *Nature* **322**, 73–7.

Lenk, U., Oexle, K., Voit, T., Ancker, U., Hellner, K.A., Speer, A., and Hubner, C. (1996). A cysteine 3 340 substitution in the dystroglycan-binding domain of dystrophin associated with Duchenne muscular dystrophy, mental retardation and absence of the ERG β-wave. *Human Molecular Genetics* **5** (7), 973–5.

McKusick, V.A. (1992). *Mendelian inheritance in man*, 10th edn. Johns Hopkins University Press, Baltimore, Maryland.

Monaco, A.P., Bertelson, C.J., Middlesworth, W., *et al.* (1985). Detection of deletions spanning the Duchenne muscular dystrophy locus using a tightly linked DNA segment. *Nature* **316**, 842–5.

Monaco, A.P., Bertelson, C.J., Liecht-Gallati, S., Moser, H., and Kunkel, L.M. (1988). An explanation for the phenotypic differences between patients bearing partial deletions of the DMD locus. *Genomics* **2**, 90–5.

Norwood, F.L.M., Sutherland-Smith, A.S., Keep, N.H., and Kendrick-Jones, J. (2000). The structure of the N-terminal actin-binding domain of human dystrophin and how mutations in this domain may cause Duchenne or Becker muscular dystrophy. *Structure* **8**, 481–91.

Pizzuti, A., Pieretti, M., Fenwick, R.G., Gibbs, R.A., and Caskey, C.T. (1992). A transposon-like element in the deletion-prone region of the dystrophin gene. *Genomics* **13** (3), 594–600.

Ray, P.N., Belfall, B., Duff, C., *et al.* (1985). Cloning of the breakpoint of an X;21 translocation associated with Duchenne muscular dystrophy. *Nature* **318**, 672–5.

Suminaga, R., Takeshima, Y., Yasuda, K., Shiga, N., Nakamura, H., and Matsuo, M. (2000). Non-homologous recombination between Alu and LINE-1 repeats caused a 430-kb deletion in the dystrophin gene: a novel source of genomic instability. *Journal of Human Genetics* **45** (6), 331–6

Worton, R.G., Duff, C., Sylvester, J.E., Schmickel, R.D., and Willard, H.F. (1984). Duchenne muscular dystrophy involving translocation of the *dmd* gene next to ribosomal RNA genes. *Science* **224**, 1447–9.

Chapter 10

Pathogenesis

When this book was first written in the mid-1980s, much space was given to an examination of the evidence for what were referred to as the vascular, neurogenic, and membrane hypotheses of causation. But, with the discovery that the primary cause was a deficiency of dystrophin located at the cell membrane, there seemed no longer any reason to consider much previous research on the subject. However, among these previous research findings, there may be important ideas necessary for a full and complete understanding of the disease process. Thus, although a vascular or neurogenic defect is definitely not the primary cause, nevertheless, the contribution of a not entirely adequate blood supply might aggravate the disease process. Proper functioning and organization of the neuromuscular junction is also essential for the correct differentiation of the muscle fibres. We do not know at the moment if such influences, in addition to a deficiency of muscle dystrophin during muscle development, might contribute to the full expression of an abnormal phenotype. With the recent advances in our understanding of the cellular partners of dystrophin, a complex pathogenic scenario of its functions has emerged. These functions will be discussed in this chapter and are summarized in Table 10.1.

Evidence in support of a mechanical role for dystrophin

Protein structure

Sequence analysis of the dystrophin gene has from the outset attributed to dystrophin a structural role. The N-terminal first ~246 amino acids of dystrophin contains the main actin-binding region, which shows significant sequence homology to a number of structural molecules that include α-actinin and spectrin. Patients with relatively small in-frame deletions in this region, for example, exons 3–13; 3–15; 4–18, often have a Duchenne muscular dystrophy (DMD) phenotype, and single exon 3 and 5 deletions (in frame) have been associated with either DMD or intermediate phenotypes. These observations, together with those made in transgenic mouse models, strongly suggest that interactions between dystrophin and the F-actin associated cytoskeleton are of considerable functional relevance (Fig. 10.1).

Table 10.1 Summary of cellular functions proposed for dystrophin in muscle

Mechanical role
Stabilization of the membrane by linking to F-actin
Force transmission

Cell signalling
Syntrophin and dystrobrevin
Grb2 (growth factor receptor bound 2), a signal-transducting adaptor protein
  (via β-dystroglycan)
Calmodulin (regulator of calcium-dependent kinases)
Serine/threonine kinases (via β2 syntrophin)
nNOS (neuronal nitric oxide synthase)

Others
Calcium homeostasis
Role in smooth muscle
GLUT 4 translocation
Regeneration and fibrosis
Immune factors
Neurogenic abnormalities

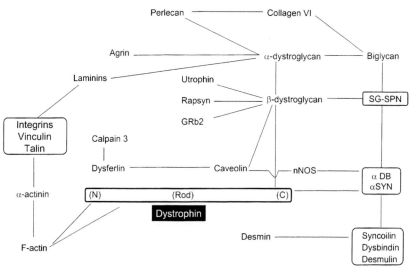

Fig. 10.1 Proposed binding interactions of various muscle proteins. (Adapted from Emery (2002).)

The *N*-terminal domain is followed by a large region consisting of 24 spectrin-like triple helical repeats that form the *rod domain*. This region of dystrophin also contains an actin-binding site (between spectrin repeats 11 and 14) that is not present in the utrophin rod domain. The functional relevance of this difference is not yet understood. Large in-frame deletions in the central rod domain are often associated with the milder Becker muscular dystrophy (BMD) suggesting that, from a functional perspective, this domain is not crucial. This has been further confirmed by the transgenic experiments with the engineering of *mdx* mice that express a construct with a deletion of exons 17–48, resulting in marked amelioration of the pathology. These observations are of considerable importance with respect to attempts to develop a gene therapy for DMD using truncated versions of dystrophin, since only very few viral vectors can carry the full-length 14 kb dystrophin cDNA, in addition to a promoter. The capacity of even shorter carefully engineered isoforms to rescue the pathological phenotype in *mdx* mice has been further assessed by Chamberlain's group using both transgenic and gene therapy approaches. The results obtained with these experiments are encouraging (Harper *et al.* 2002).

Immediately after the rod domain is the *WW domain*, which separates the rod from the *cysteine-rich* domain. The WW is a motif found in several proteins with regulatory and signalling functions. This region is involved in the interaction of dystrophin with β-dystroglycan. This link is critical as deletions or missense mutations in the cysteine-rich domain of dystrophin that eliminate β-dystroglycan binding cause DMD. At least part of the reason for this may be that β-dystroglycan binds α-dystroglycan, a highly glycosylated receptor for laminin α2 chain and other proteins, thereby mediating a link between the cytoskeleton and the extracellular matrix.

The cysteine-rich domain contains sequence motifs involved in various interactions. These are two EF-hand motifs (involved in Ca^{2+} binding), followed by a ZZ domain that binds to calmodulin in a Ca^{2+} dependent manner. Adjacent to the cysteine-rich domain is an alternatively spliced region and two coiled-coil motifs that form the *C*-terminus of dystrophin. The alternatively spliced region binds syntrophin, while the coiled-coil motifs bind dystrobrevin. This coiled-coils region is arranged in an α-helical manner, similarly to the rod domain. The cellular functions of dystrobrevin and syntrophin have yet to be established. However, various lines of evidence suggest that these molecules are involved in cell signalling. In particular, syntrophin binds to neuronal nitric oxide synthase (nNOS), sodium channels, stress-activated protein kinase-3, and a microtubule-associated serine/threonine kinase.

Localization of dystrophin

Dystrophin is not distributed evenly on the inner side of the sarcolemma, but appears to be enriched at the neuromuscular and myotendinous junctions and the costamers.

The *costamers* were first described in 1983 as discrete subsarcolemmal vinculin-rich domains that flank the Z-disc and link the contractile apparatus to the sarcolemma along the entire length of the fibre. They have since been shown to be composed of a number of cytoskeletal proteins that include dystrophin, talin, spectrin, ankyrin, and desmin. This arrangement facilitates the lateral transmission of force and alignment of the sarcomers, which may be particularly relevant to fibres that do not run from one end of the muscle to the other but rather terminate in the perimysium.

At the *neuromuscular junction* the muscle fibre membrane is thrown into a series of folds, with the crests of each fold adjacent to the nerve terminal and containing the acetylcholine receptors. Dystrophin and utrophin occupy distinct domains within this region with dystrophin and the voltage-gated sodium channels being found at the base of each fold and utrophin co-localizing with the acetylcholine receptors at the crests. The muscle fibre membrane is also highly folded at the myotendinous junction. A comparison of *mdx* mice with those deficient in α7–β1 integrin suggests that that, whilst integrin α7 is the major receptor connecting the muscle cell to the tendon, the dystrophin–glycoprotein complex is necessary for the lateral integrity of the muscle cell in this region. In the absence of dystrophin at the myotendinous junction, other cytoskeletal proteins such as talin and vinculin are upregulated.

Membrane hypothesis

It is difficult to be sure when the idea that a significant defect in DMD might reside in the muscle cell membrane was first considered. Certainly this possibility was put forward in the 1950s when several muscle enzymes were found to be increased in the serum of affected boys. Further evidence came in the mid-1970s when electron microscopy identified sarcolemmal defects in the muscle of children with DMD (the so-called delta lesions). More recently, numerous studies have shown that dystrophin-deficient *mdx* mouse muscle fibres display an increased permeability to injected macromolecules such as Procion Orange and Evans Blue, a property that is made significantly worse if the muscle has been previously subjected to eccentric contractions.

Such work clearly identifies an increased susceptibility to dystrophic membrane damage relative to normal muscle. The observation that dystrophin-deficient mouse myotubes and muscle fibres appear to be more susceptible to osmotic damage and display a substantial reduction in cortical stiffness relative to controls further supports this view.

The tensile strength of the muscle fibre surface membrane may be estimated either by measuring the suction required to burst membrane patches or by the aspiration of sarcolemmal vesicles into a micropipette of uniform bore. Using this methodology the maximum tension sustainable by normal mouse sarcolemma is only slightly higher than that for dystrophin-deficient *mdx* mice and such differences have been thought to be too small to account for the apparent increased osmotic fragility of dystrophin-deficient *mdx* fibres. This suggests that dystrophin may act to prevent membrane damage by maintaining the normal folding and organization of the sarcolemma rather than through a direct effect on tensile strength.

Linkage with the extracellular matrix

α-Dystroglycan and integrin $\alpha7$ are the two main receptors for laminin $\alpha2$ in striated muscle (see Fig. 10.1). Integrin $\alpha7$ is upregulated in DMD and *mdx* muscle. The transgenic overexpression of integrin $\alpha7$ in mice deficient in both dystrophin and utrophin results in the amelioration of some aspects of their phenotype and prolongation of their life-span. These observations emphasize the importance of maintaining a linkage between the basement membrane and the cytoskeleton of the muscle fibre. A number of transgenic experiments in several different animal models support this concept. For example, the high expression of an utrophin transgene in *mdx* mice almost totally restores normal muscle function. The overexpression of an agrin minigene in the *dy/dy* mouse, which is deficient in laminin $\alpha2$, leads to an amelioration of the dystrophic phenotype by the stabilization of α-dystroglycan and laminin $\alpha4$ and $\alpha5$ chains. Finally, the overexpression at the sarcolemma of the enzyme CT GalNAc transferase, normally located in the synapses, induces an increased expression of dystroglycan, utrophin, and other components of the dystrophin-associated protein complex at the muscle fibre. The upregulation at the sarcolemma of these synaptic proteins significantly reduces the muscle pathology of *mdx* mice.

Evidence in support of a signalling role for dystrophin

Dystrophin is part of a complex of glycoproteins (dystrophin-associated glycoprotein complex, or DAPC), some of which have been shown to have a clear signalling role. Since several of these proteins are significantly affected by dystrophin deficiency, and some have also been primarily involved in other muscular dystrophies, it is conceivable that their secondary deficiency in DMD is involved in disease pathogenesis. The proteins more closely associated to the DAPC are shown in Fig. 10.1.

For example, β-dystroglycan binds to Grb2 (growth factor receptor bound 2), a 25 kDa protein that participates in signal transduction pathways involving receptor tyrosine kinases. Many of the signalling pathways associated with the integrin axis also involve Grb2, raising the possibility that some of the signalling pathways activated by the integrins may be shared by dystroglycan.

Caveolin 3, the protein whose deficiency causes a form of autosomal dominant limb girdle muscular dystrophy (LGMD1C; see Chapter 2), has been shown to compete with dystrophin for the β-dystroglycan binding site. Mice overexpressing caveolin 3 show an apparent downregulation of dystrophin and β dystroglycan together with more severe pathological changes than those normally observed in *mdx* mice. Overall, these observations imply that the interaction between dystrophin and dystroglycan is likely to be highly dynamic.

Syntrophin also possesses the capacity to bind to Grb2 in addition to voltage-gated Na^+ channels, neuronal nitric oxide synthase (nNOS), and stress-activated protein kinase-3 (SAPK3). The dynamics of the syntrophin–dystrophin interactions appear to be regulated by calmodulin and by the phosphorylation or dephosphorylation of dystrophin. Syntrophin itself is phosphorylated by a calcium-calmodulin-dependent protein kinase that regulates its binding to dystrophin, and by stress-activated protein kinase-3 (SAPK-3). Mice deficient in α1-syntrophin display abnormalities of the neuromuscular junction with secondary reductions of utrophin, acetylcholine receptor, and acetylcholinesterase, emphasizing the importance of syntrophins in recruiting and stabilizing proteins involved in signalling at the sarcolemma. Dystrophin also has several potential phosphorylation sites in the *C*-terminal region and is the target of a variety of kinases, including calmodulin-dependent protein kinase II, p44[erk1] mitogen-activated protein kinase (MAPK), p34[cdc2] kinase, and casein kinase. The phosphorylation of dystrophin has been found to alter its affinity both for actin and syntrophin *in vitro*. While the functional significance of these phosphorylation events *in vivo* still has to be demonstrated, nonetheless they do provide possible mechanisms by which the dystrophin–glycoprotein complex can be dynamically regulated.

The *dystrobrevins* are a family of dystrophin-related proteins with homology to the *C*-terminal region of dystrophin. The presence of several tyrosine kinase consensus sites in the *C*-terminal region of certain dystrobrevin isoforms suggests that protein–protein interactions may be modulated by tyrosine phosphorylation. Further evidence in favour of a role for the dystrobrevins in cell signalling comes from the α-dystrobrevin knock-out mouse, which develops a mild dystrophy but fails to show any overt disruption of the dystrophin-associated glycoprotein complex. A possible mutation in the α1 dystrobrevin gene has been found in a single family with dilated cardiomyopathy. Further mutations will have to be identified before definitively assigning a role for α1 dystrobrevin in dilated cardiomyopathy.

Secondary deficiency of nNOS: modulation of blood flow and immune response

Dystrobrevin binds to the *C*-terminus of dystrophin and together with syntrophin forms a ternary complex that is responsible for localizing nNOS to the muscle fibre membrane. DMD patients and *mdx* mice fail to localize nNOS to the membrane. Mice in which the genes for either α1 dystrobrevin or α1 syntrophin have been knocked out also fail to properly localize nNOS. However, only the α1 dystrobrevin knock-out animals display any signs of a muscular dystrophy. Since no gross histological changes are evident in either α1 syntrophin or nNOS knock-out mice, the membrane localization of nNOS was initially not considered to be an important factor in the pathogenesis of DMD. However, sympathetic nervous input to the muscular vasculature causes vasoconstriction that is modulated differently in muscle at rest and during exercise. Various lines of evidence now indicate that the inhibition of sympathetic vasoconstriction in contracting muscle is defective in mice with a deficiency of nNOS at the sarcolemma. An abnormal regulation of blood flow within exercising skeletal muscle has also been documented in DMD patients. The vasoconstrictor response (measured as a decrease in muscle oxygenation) to reflex sympathetic activation is not attenuated during exercise of dystrophic muscles. In contrast, this protective mechanism is intact in healthy children and other disease controls in whom there is no loss of nNOS from the membrane. These observations are of particular interest when considering that necrosis often takes place in groups of fibres in both *mdx* mice and DMD patients, a feature that has often been interpreted as indicative of ischaemia and thus a possible vascular problem.

Other dystrophin functions

Calcium homeostasis

The possibility that increased intracellular calcium might be a significant factor in the pathogenesis of DMD was put forward more than 20 years ago. The reason for this increase was unclear although it was recognized that increased intracellular calcium could account for muscle necrosis through the enhancement of calcium-activated proteases. Various techniques (histochemical, biochemical, and electron microscopic) seemingly supported this by showing that the total calcium content was elevated in muscle in DMD, even from a very early age (see Chapter 4), as well as in BMD. Whilst these features were not specific to dystrophin-deficient muscle, early studies suggested these to be more severe in DMD compared to other neuromuscular disorders. A significant increase in the number of calcium-positive fibres in male fetuses at-risk for DMD has also been reported.

Not all of these earlier studies, however, could distinguish the intracellular component of the total calcium. This could only be accomplished several years later following significant methodological advances. With the advent of fluorescent indicators it became possible to measure free intracellular calcium $[Ca^{2+}]_i$ and so to evaluate the calcium dynamics of dystrophin-deficient muscle fibres and myotubes *in vitro*. Unfortunately, rather than clarifying the situation, the results obtained so far have proved to be controversial. At least part of the reason for this may be secondary to subtle methodological differences among the techniques used or the preparation of the tissues. For example, muscle fibre preparation or culture conditions can vary markedly between laboratories and this might affect results. Furthermore, all the evidence suggests that dystrophin function relies on the maintenance of a link between the cytoskeleton and the extracellular matrix, and isolated fibres and cultured muscle may not prove to be entirely reliable models in which to evaluate the role of the dystrophin axis on $[Ca^{2+}]_i$ handling. It should also be noted that, as a consequence of the behaviour of the fluorescent indicators themselves, it has not been possible to measure $[Ca^{2+}]_i$ immediately under the membrane, which would seem to be most relevant in the case of dystrophin deficiency. Nonetheless, attempts to overcome this have been made recently by using plasma membrane calcium-activated K^+ channels as subsarcolemmal calcium probes. This work suggests that in the absence of dystrophin there is, in fact, a higher subsarcolemmal concentration of $[Ca^{2+}]_i$. The development of membrane-localizing fluorescent probes for $[Ca^{2+}]_i$ should enable this aspect to be further investigated in the future.

Another line of enquiry has included the analysis of sequestered calcium using organelle-specific probes. Skeletal muscle is necessarily efficient at controlling large transient fluctuations in $[Ca^{2+}]_i$, and any abnormal influx in calcium may be rapidly sequestered into intracellular compartments such as the mitochondria. This is supported by the observation that the mitochondria of *mdx* myotubes show greater increases in Ca^{2+} following potassium chloride-induced depolarization than controls. Interestingly, these differences were found to precede alterations in either the cytosol or the cytoplasmic region beneath the membrane, which themselves only became significant at a later stage of myotube differentiation. Taking into account the key role played by mitochondrial Ca^{2+} handling in cell death, these data suggest that mitochondria are potential targets of impaired Ca^{2+} homeostasis in muscular dystrophy. Indeed, this may explain why alterations in cytosolic calcium are not always evident despite the wealth of data from electrophysiological measurements that indicates an increase in calcium leak activity, particularly within the vicinity of artificially induced membrane tears. Since the activity of these channels is apparently decreased in the presence of leupeptin, a protease inhibitor, these observations lend weight to the hypothesis that an initial influx of calcium due perhaps to transient membrane damage leads to an increase in calcium-activated proteases. These proteases then induce further

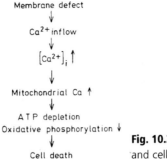

Membrane defect
↓
Ca^{2+} inflow
↓
$[Ca^{2+}]_i$ ↑
↓
Mitochondrial Ca ↑
↓
ATP depletion
Oxidative phosphorylation ↓
↓
Cell death

Fig. 10.2 Calcium influx and cell death.

Ca^{2+} influx by acting upon Ca^{2+} leak channels, the result of which is a mitochondrial overload, reduction in oxidative phosphorylation, and cell death (Fig. 10.2).

In summary, therefore, the dystrophin-deficient muscle has, on average, increased calcium content that can be demonstrated with methodologies that are able to measure macromolecular concentrations of calcium.

Calcium content in the cytosol of dystrophin-deficient muscle (non-necrotic fibres) is not grossly abnormal. Calcium might, however, be accumulated in different subcellular compartments such as just beneath the sarcolemma and in the mitochondria.

Whatever the mechanism, the accumulation of calcium (either as a result of specific calcium homeostasis or as a consequences of generalized and gross sarcolemmal damage following contraction), there then follows enhancement of calcium-activated proteases as well as mitochondrial overload, resulting in a reduction in oxidative phosphorylation and eventually cell death (Fig. 10.2).

Role in smooth muscle

Dystrophin is specifically localized in the caveolae-rich domains of the smooth muscle sarcolemma together with caveolin. This raises the possibility that the absence of dystrophin in DMD might result in some form of vascular dysfunction. Evidence of abnormalities in the peripheral circulation initially came from early work performed in the 1960s and 1970s by Démos and colleagues in Paris. Since then it has been found that functional abnormalities of the system are implied by the increased blood loss in children with DMD undergoing spinal surgery. However, detailed studies on the vascular reactivity of dystrophin-deficient *mdx* mice suggest no defect with the exception of flow-induced dilatation (shear stress), which is decreased by 50–60 per cent. It has been hypothesized that dystrophin could play a specific role in shear-stress mechanotransduction in arterial endothelial cells.

Further abnormalities in muscle blood flow have been associated with a deficiency in nNOS (see above).

GLUT4 translocation

Dystrophin contains actin-binding sites at its *N*-terminus and the distribution of F-actin is significantly abnormal as a result of dystrophin deficiency in the mouse, although such studies have not yet been performed in human muscle. This may be of considerable function relevance as one interesting role of the actin cytoskeleton is the recycling of the glucose transporter GLUT4 between the cytoplasm and sarcolemma. GLUT4 co-localizes with dystrophin and various studies have demonstrated a deficiency of GLUT4 at the sarcolemma of skeletal and cardiac muscle in the absence of dystrophin. This observation is paralleled by the biochemical finding of a reduction in glucose transport in hearts of *mdx* mice. Furthermore, magnetic spectroscopic data have demonstrated an *in vivo* glycolytic defect in both *mdx* dystrophic mice and patients with dystrophin deficiency. The role of abnormal glucose metabolism in the muscle degeneration seen in DMD is likely to be limited but perhaps still significant. These observations highlight an important point, namely, that proteins with an obvious structural role may also indirectly contribute to metabolic function.

Regeneration and fibrosis

Myogenic proliferation and differentiation is under the control of growth factors such as transforming growth factor β (TGF-β), insulin-like growth factors (IGFs) and basic fibroblast growth factor (bFGF). In DMD the chronic accumulation of sclerotic scar tissue in the interstitial space of skeletal muscle is attributed to secondary pathological processes and may itself assume a pathogenic role and contribute to disease progression by interfering with effective muscle regeneration and re-innervation. bFGF enhances the proliferation of skeletal muscle cells *in vitro*, and elevated levels have been reported in the serum of some patients with DMD. bFGF has also been shown to be elevated in necrotic and regenerating muscle fibres of the *mdx* mouse and dystrophin-deficient cats (hypertrophic feline muscular dystrophy, HFMD) where it has been linked to efficient regeneration. This increase is less striking in DMD patients and dystrophic dogs, although whether it accounts for the markedly different phenotypes seen between the two species remains to be demonstrated.

Insulin-like growth factor I (IGF-I) has also been shown to stimulate satellite cell proliferation although its main function is the induction of muscle differentiation. *mdx* mice carrying a transgene for IGF-1 display a reduction in fibrosis (diaphragm) and necrosis, and an increase in muscle mass and force generation relative to age-matched *mdx* mice. The overexpression of an IGF-1 transgene has also been reported to ameliorate the early histopathological changes in the *mdx* mouse. These observations underscore the role of growth factors in mediating efficient muscle fibre regeneration. The fact that fibrosis only occurs in DMD and the dystrophic dog but not in the dystrophic cat or *mdx* mouse, raises some important questions regarding pathogenetic mechanisms in these different species (Chapter 7, p. 129).

Immune factors

The degeneration of muscle fibres in DMD is associated with an invasion of inflammatory cells such as macrophages and T-lymphocytes raising the possibility that fibre necrosis may be accentuated by T-cell-mediated injury as occurs in polymyositis. It has further been suggested that altered expression of extracellular matrix ligands and receptors may promote cytotoxic lymphocytes to recognize self as foreign (non-self) and attack the muscle membrane, which then results in the ingress of complement and calcium with subsequent fibre necrosis. A significant increase in the number of T suppressor/cytotoxic cells in the peripheral blood in DMD supports this hypothesis. Furthermore, it has been found that HLA class I antigens (MHC I) are expressed in skeletal muscle in various muscular dystrophies but not in normal muscle. This would render the dystrophic muscle more susceptible to T-cell-mediated attack and membrane damage in addition to any mechanical damage consequent on a defective cytoskeleton. The overexpression of MHC class I antigens is clearly not limited to X-linked dystrophies but represents an epiphenomenon. Nevertheless, it seems reasonable that the expression of a surface antigen that then renders the cell susceptible to T-cell attack has a number of important implications.

Mast cells play a prominent role in inflammation and have been shown to be concentrated in areas of muscle fibre regeneration and necrosis. It has been suggested that the proteolytic activity of mast cells may be responsible for the simultaneous degeneration of large groups of fibres seen in the *mdx* mouse (grouped fibre necrosis). Dystrophin-deficient muscle is clearly more susceptible to muscle fibre necrosis when exposed to intramuscular injections of purified mast cell granules and an exaggerated pathology is found in *mdx* mice with a heightened mast cell activity. Moreover, a strong correlation between mast cell content and localization, and the clinico-histopathological progression in humans, dogs, and mice has been previously demonstrated. Additional data in support of the role of immune cells in promoting the pathology observed in dystrophin-deficient muscle comes from the observation of increased numbers of activated dendritic cells in dystrophic muscle relative to controls that mediate immune responses and probably induce micro-environmental changes.

Another relevant immune factor is NO; this molecule also has an anti-inflammatory and cytoprotective function, and thus its loss from dystrophic muscle could exacerbate muscle inflammation and fibre damage by inflammatory cells. Recent work supports this by showing that the transgenic expression of NOS is able to ameliorate muscular dystrophy in the *mdx* mice. Expression of the NOS transgene in *mdx* muscle also prevented the majority of muscle membrane injury that is detectable *in vivo*, and resulted in large decreases in serum creatine kinase (SCK) concentrations. The significance of this is shown by the additional finding that *mdx* muscle macrophages are cytolytic only at the elevated concentrations they are present in dystrophic, nNOS-deficient muscle.

Antibody-mediated depletion of macrophages from *mdx* mice also causes a significant reduction in muscle membrane injury. These findings suggest that macrophages promote injury of dystrophin-deficient muscle, and the loss of normal levels of NO production by dystrophic muscle exacerbates inflammation and membrane injury.

Neurogenic abnormalities

In addition to muscle, dystrophin is also expressed in some neurons and there is now no doubt that its deficiency in these cells affects the central nervous system and is responsible for some degree of mental retardation (Chapter 6, p. 101 et seq.). The question we are concerned with here, however, is the possibility that defects at the neuromuscular junction may adversely affect muscle innervation. Many characteristics of fast and slow muscles, including their enzyme profiles and physiological properties, are dependent on appropriate innervation. Furthermore, animal models clearly show that dystroglycan, dystrophin, utrophin, and dystrobrevin are all required for the normal postnatal maturation of the neuromuscular junction. Abnormalities at the neuromuscular junction in the form of focal atrophy of the postsynaptic regions have previously been documented in DMD. However, despite these areas of focal degeneration the amplitude and frequency of miniature end-plate potentials following nerve stimulation appear normal. In summary, therefore, while subtle defects of the neuromuscular junction might well exist, their role in disease pathogenesis remains to be clarified.

Gene profiling

Using cDNA derived from DMD muscle and hybridizing this on a microarray of DNA sequences of known (and some unknown) genes, it has been found that the transcription of several hundred genes appears to be altered in DMD (Porter *et al.* 2002, Noguchi *et al.* 2003). A large number of the observed changes might well have been expected from what is already known of the biochemical changes in dystrophic muscle (Chapter 7). Nevertheless, this approach does offer an opportunity to possibly identify unknown genes whose transcriptional activity is changed in DMD, and some of these might prove to be significant in the pathogenesis of DMD.

Conclusions

The primary defect in DMD is a deficiency of dystrophin, the consequences of which are most profound in striated muscle. Dystrophin is a key member of the dystrophin–glycoprotein complex that, when disrupted, leads to an increase in muscle fibre membrane fragility. This is thought to result in an abnormal influx of calcium leading to subsequent fibre degeneration. However, additional mechanisms are likely to play a significant role in the pathogenesis of DMD, including defective glucose utilization, blunted vascular response following exercise, increased susceptibility to cytokines, and aberrant cell signalling, the details of which remain to be clarified. Based on current information, a tentative scheme of the possible pathogenetic pathways in DMD has been drawn up (Fig. 10.3). However, such a scheme, though it may concentrate the mind, gives no indication as to the primary cause of the pattern of progressive muscle weakness, and why there is marked differential muscle involvement. The major challenge for the future will be to untangle

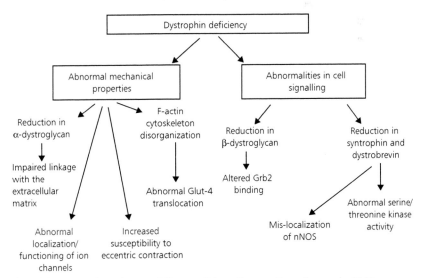

Fig. 10.3 A tentative scheme of the possible pathogenetic pathways in DMD.

some of the pathways that give rise to the characteristic pattern of pathogenesis and so open up the prospect of some form of therapy into this seriously debilitating disease.

References and further reading

Anderson, L.V.B. (2002). Dystrophinopathies. In *Structural and molecular basis of skeletal muscle diseases* (ed. G. Karpati), pp. 6–19. ISN Neuropath Press, Basel.

Blake, D.J., Weir, A., Newey, S.E., and Davies, K.E. (2002). Function and genetics of dystrophin and dystrophin-related proteins in muscle. *Physiological Review* 82 (2), 291–329.

Burton, E.A. and Davies, K.E. (2001). The pathogenesis of Duchenne muscular dystrophy. In *Pathogenesis of neurodegenerative disorders* (ed. M.P. Mattson), pp. 239–84. Humana Press, Totowa, New Jersey.

Emery, A.E.H. (2002). Muscular dystrophy into the new millennium. *Neuromuscular Disorders* 12, 343–9.

Harper, S.Q., Hauser, M.A., DelloRusso, C., Duan, D., Crawford, R.W., Phelps, S.F., Harper, H.A., Robinson, A.S., Engelhardt, J.F., Brooks, S.V., and Chamberlain, J.S. (2002). Modular flexibility of dystrophin: implications for gene therapy of Duchenne muscular dystrophy. *Nat Med* 8, 253–61.

Noguchi, S., Tsukahara, T., Fujita, M. *et al.* (2003). cDNA microarray analysis of individual Duchenne muscular dystrophy patients. *Human Molecular Genetics* 12, 595–600.

O'Brien, K.F. and Kunkel, L.M. (2001). Dystrophin and muscular dystrophy: past, present, and future. *Molecular Genetics and Metabolism* 74 (1–2), 75–88.

Porter, J.D., Khanna, S., Kaminski, H.J., Rao, J.S., Merriam, A.P., Richmonds, C.R., Leahy, P., Li, J., Guo, W., and Andrade, F.H. (2002). A chronic inflammatory response dominates the skeletal muscle molecular signature in dystrophin-deficient mdx muscle. *Human Molecular Genetics* 11, 263–72.

Rando, T.A. (2001). The dystrophin–glycoprotein complex, cellular signaling, and the regulation of cell survival in the muscular dystrophies. *Muscle and Nerve* 24 (12), 1575–94.

Chapter 11

Prevention

Since Duchenne muscular dystrophy (DMD) is a serious disorder for which at present there is no effective treatment, a great deal of emphasis has been given to prevention. This involves the ascertainment of women likely to have an affected son and the provision of genetic counselling and prenatal diagnosis for such women.

Ascertainment of families at risk

The ascertainment of women at risk of having an affected child is the first pre-requisite of prevention. Logically, this would seem best achieved by screening all females to determine which ones are likely to be carriers. This is impractical, however, because there is as yet no simple test that could be used to detect all carriers and, in any event, such screening would be prohibitively expensive. Furthermore, as already observed, in roughly one-third of cases the mother is not a carrier, the affected son being the result of a new mutation (see Chapter 8).

Another approach might be to screen all pregnancies for affected males. However, quite apart from technical and economic considerations, this would raise a number of serious ethical problems, which were discussed in Chapter 8. At present, the only practical solution is to ensure that all affected boys in the community are ascertained as early as possible, and that their mothers, and subsequently other female relatives, are then tested to determine their carrier status and the likelihood of the disorder recurring.

Population screening

Because SCK levels in affected boys are grossly elevated from birth, there is the potential for detection in the neonatal period (see Chapter 8). This can be achieved by determining the serum creatine kinase (SCK) level in dried blood spots obtained from a heel prick. The blood spots are placed on a filter paper card and the air-dried specimen can then be assayed immediately or stored. Enzyme activity remains stable for several weeks at room temperature provided direct heat and sunlight are avoided. Specimens can therefore be conveniently sent by post. With this technique it is possible to screen newborns for Duchenne and other forms of muscular dystrophy (a child affected by merosin-deficient congenital muscular dystrophy was, for example, identified as part of one of the pilot screening programmes for DMD) but this technique does not screen for female carriers.

The false positive rate with the various methods of SCK determination ranges between 0.02 and 0.40 (Table 8.2, p. 134). When a serum sample yields a grossly elevated SCK level, the diagnosis has to be confirmed by appropriate investigations. There will always be some false positives with this test because it has to be sufficiently sensitive to detect all cases. It seems likely, therefore, that the false negative rate among those tested will be low, and only limited to laboratory or administrative errors or failure to test an infant who subsequently develops the disease.

However, the important question remains as to whether such screening is really justified. It can be argued that, if an affected boy were detected sufficiently early and his mother proved to be a carrier and was counselled, second cases in the family might be prevented. It has been estimated that up to 15–20 per cent of cases might be prevented in this way. In a series of our patients for whom precise information was available, there were 67 families in which an affected boy was born but at the time no one else was affected in the family and the mother subsequently became pregnant. The average time between the birth of this son and the birth of the next child was 2.71 years (SD, 1.45; range, 1.0–7.0 years). Thus the next pregnancy was conceived on average less than 2 years after the birth of a son *who subsequently proved to be affected*. Since at least 75 per cent of affected boys present suspicious signs after this age and the mean age at diagnosis is around 5 years of age with a range of 2–8 years, most parents would have been completely unaware of the risks in the next pregnancy. In fact, 10 sons in the next or a following pregnancy subsequently proved to be affected.

Neonatal screening has also been justified on financial grounds, it being argued that the tests are relatively cheap to carry out and prevention compared with management would be cost-effective. It could also be combined with neonatal screening for other genetic disorders such as cystic fibrosis.

Finally, most parents of affected boys questioned in a survey appeared to favour such screening for a number of reasons.

- It would prevent the anxiety that results from the long delays and unfounded reassurances often experienced between the first symptoms and the establishment of the diagnosis.
- Parents have a 'right' to know as soon as possible.
- It would help prevent further affected children.
- It has practical advantages in affording an early opportunity to obtain appropriate housing, for example.
- There are emotional advantages.

However, those questioned in this study were all parents who had already had an affected son. The concern is of presenting a couple with the devastating news that their newborn son has a serious genetic disorder when they are completely unprepared for this. Furthermore, the parents have to cope with the problem some 4 or 5 years sooner than they would otherwise have had to. Some have therefore advocated a compromise, that screening might be restricted to those boys who are not walking by the age of 18 months, or when there is a delay in motor and mental development for no obvious reason. The age of 18 months was selected because by this time almost all normal boys have learned to walk but only about 50 per cent of affected boys. It has been reasoned that this more restricted screening would have the advantages of involving fewer tests (and therefore lower costs), and that the results would be easier to interpret and less likely to cause anxiety because the parents' concern is already aroused. Of course, since the screening would be carried out later, fewer secondary cases (less than 10 per cent) could be prevented. It would therefore be less effective. It would also be necessary to establish procedures for informing all family doctors of the requirement for testing and the referral of blood samples to an appropriate centre. This could present organizational difficulties.

However the subject is viewed, screening for DMD has so far failed to generate a great deal of enthusiasm either among paediatricians or geneticists. There is little doubt, however, that when an effective treatment eventually becomes available interest will be rekindled. For it seems probable that the sooner any treatment is begun the more likely it is to be effective and arrest the course of the disease. A number of issues will then have to be faced including the very careful and sensitive counselling of parents of proven positive cases.

At present most paediatricians and geneticists confine their activities to the family of an affected boy. All of his female relatives can be screened in order to assess their carrier status, and records of those found to be at risk can be maintained on a confidential register system for subsequent follow-up.

Carrier detection

The whole problem of genetic counselling in DMD revolves around the detection of female carriers. If all mothers of affected boys were carriers, the situation would be much simpler. This is, however, not the case in approximately one-third of cases and, in any event, the carrier status of sisters and daughters of carrier mothers often has to be determined.

Definition of carrier status

First it is necessary to consider the definition of a carrier. In the past, confusion on this point has often led to difficulties in interpreting the results of any proposed tests for detecting carriers. There are three accepted categories of carriers based on genetic considerations.

1   Definite (or obligate) carriers who are mothers of an affected son but who also have an affected brother, affected nephew by their sister, or an affected maternal uncle or other maternal male relative. Included in this category are also mothers of affected sons by different non-consanguineous fathers.

2   Probable carriers who are mothers with two or more affected sons but with no other affected relatives. This could be the result of germ-line mosaicism (see later) or autosomal recessive limb girdle muscular dystrophy of childhood which clinically resembles DMD.

3   Possible carriers who are mothers of an isolated case as well as their sisters and other female relatives. This category also includes female relatives of definite and probable carriers. The probability of all such women being carriers has to be determined. The term 'suspected carrier' is frequently used for any woman who is at risk of being a carrier.

Biological considerations

The evaluation of carrier detection tests has been bedevilled by several factors. Some of these are inherent in that, DMD being an X-linked recessive disorder, there will inevitably be variability in expression in carrier females because of random inactivation of the X chromosome. This means that a proportion of carriers is unlikely to be detectable by any biochemical or histochemical methods except one employing cloned cells to identify two populations or one based on DNA studies. If a subsequent pregnancy is terminated it may be possible to confirm the diagnosis by studying the aborted fetus. If the fetus is found to be affected, it could confirm the carrier status of the mother.

Methodological considerations

Even though the cause of DMD is now known and abnormalities of muscle dystrophin and DNA are detectable in some carriers, we shall see that this is not always so. The advent of DNA markers for carrier detection has, however, made other approaches to the problem redundant. Some of these other approaches will, however, be discussed as a mutation may not be available in all families (that is, at least 20–30 per cent of cases of DMD or Becker muscular dystrophy (BMD) do not carry easily identifiable mutations).

It should also be remembered that a proportion of carriers may exhibit some degree of muscle weakness—so-called 'manifesting carriers' (see Chapter 5, p. 83 et seq.).

Carrier detection tests

There are essentially three approaches used to detect carriers: SCK, muscle pathology including immunocytochemistry, and DNA analysis.

Serum creatine kinase

For many years the most widely used single test for detecting carriers was the SCK level. Following the introduction in clinical practice of the test by Schapira and colleagues in 1960, the detection rate obtained by a number of investigators in the following years was around 60–70 per cent, and has not changed significantly since. Its great advantage is its simplicity. Furthermore, the results can be combined with data from linkage analysis to provide valuable additional information for carrier detection. However, in applying the test, possible causes of variation both in female controls and carriers must be considered. This variability is partly biological in origin. A slight rise in activity over the course of the day, and slightly higher levels in summer compared with winter have been reported. However, both diurnal and seasonal variations are small and from a practical point of view are relatively unimportant.

The stage of the menstrual cycle and the use of oral contraception have little effect on the SCK level, but vigorous exercise may cause significant increases though normal daily activity is without any material effect. Age also has to be considered. Several studies have indicated that levels are significantly higher in teenage (especially premenarchal) girls compared with adult women. Pregnancy is also an important factor, levels being significantly lower in the early stages and significantly higher immediately postpartum, where the latter is presumably due to the release of enzymes from the involuting myometrium.

Racial factors may also be involved since the mean level in Black females has been found to be significantly greater than in Caucasian females in the USA.

All these various factors also have an effect on SCK levels in carriers. Standardized exercise (on a walking machine or a bicycle ergometer) has been claimed by some to accentuate SCK levels in carriers more than controls provided that it is strenuous and the effects are followed for several hours afterwards. It has therefore been recommended as a provocative test in suspected carriers with a borderline SCK level.

Some studies have suggested that carrier detection might be better in childhood but, among daughters of definite carriers who are aged 15 and over and who have not yet had any children, the proportion with SCK levels exceeding the normal 95 percentile (86 IU) for adult women was not significantly different from the expected proportion (31.20 per cent) based on the findings in definite carriers (Table 11.1).

SCK levels in carriers may also be affected by genetic factors. This problem has been examined by considering correlations between SCK levels in various female relatives within families of definite carriers (Table 11.2). All the correlations were positive but none was significantly different from zero. If there are any familial similarities in SCK levels these would therefore seem to be relatively unimportant.

In view of the various technical and biological variations that may influence SCK levels, it is therefore not surprising that there is a considerable spread of values in controls, the distribution being positively skewed. In carriers the spread is even greater and the distribution even more skewed, but there is no suggestion of any bimodality (Fig. 11.1). Since the distributions in the two groups are so different, results have been expressed as the ratio (h) of normal homozygosity (Y_1) to

Table 11.1 The proportion of daughters of definite carriers who have SCK levels that exceed the normal 95 percentile (86 IU) for adult women (unpublished data)

	Number	Age (years)			Proportion	
		Range	Mean	SD	Number	%
Controls	200	18–52	27.06	9.10	11	5.50
Carriers	125	17–70	41.69	11.67	78	62.40
Controls	65	15–20	18.72	0.67	3	4.62
Daughters of carriers	49	15–20	17.33	1.84	16	32.65
	72	15–39	19.78	4.64	21	29.17

Table 11.2 Correlations between SCK levels in females within families of definite carriers. The correlations between sisters (daughters of definite carriers) refer to: (1) all sisters; (2) sisters where at least two sisters in a family had SCK levels in excess of 170 IU and are therefore likely to be carriers; or (3) sisters where at least two sisters in a family had SCK levels less than 86 IU and are therefore unlikely to be carriers (unpublished data)

	Carrier mothers and daughters	Daughters of carriers		
		Sisters (1)	Sisters (2)	Sisters (3)
Number	101	111	20	41
Correlation	0.016	0.138	0.182	0.112
Students 't'	0.158	1.455	0.785	0.704

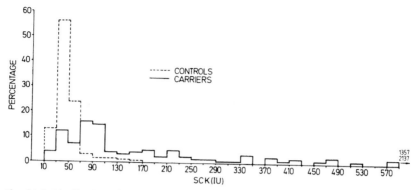

Fig. 11.1 Distribution of SCK levels determined under standardized conditions in 200 normal adult control females and 125 definite carriers.

Table 11.3 Distribution of SCK levels in controls and carriers (unpublished data)

SCK (IU)	Controls		Carriers h		(Y_1/Y_2)
	Number	% (Y_1)	Number	% (Y_2)	
11–30	26	13.0	5	4.0	3.25
31–50	112	56.0	15	12.0	4.67
51–70	47	23.5	9	7.2	3.26
71–90	6	3.0	20	16.0	0.19
91–110	3	1.5	18	14.4	0.10
111–170	6	3.0	14	11.2	—
>170	0	0.0	44	35.2	—
Total	200	100.0	125	100.0	—

heterozygosity (Y_2) as in Table 11.3. The normal 95 percentile (based on the cumulative distribution curve) is 86 IU. Seventy-eight (62 per cent) of definite carriers had levels that exceeded this, and 44 (35 per cent) had levels outside the upper limit of the normal range of 170 IU.

Because of the variability in SCK levels in carriers, our practice and that of others has been, where possible, to take the mean of samples obtained on three separate occasions in the belief that this might provide a better guide to carrier status. However, compared with the values obtained with single determinations in controls, no matter how the upper limit of normal is defined, repeat testing seems to have little overall effect on the discriminatory value of the test (Table 11.4).

Table 11.4 Proportion (%) of carriers (N = 94) with SCK levels that exceed the normal upper limit depending on whether the first, mean, or highest of three determinations is used

	95 percentile (86 IU)	Median × 2.5 (110 IU)	Median × 3 (132 IU)
First	58	49	40
Mean	64	46	40
Highest	65	52	41
Controls	5	3	1

Muscle pathology

Different types of abnormalities can be found in the muscle biopsy of carriers, which range from gross morphological changes to subtle abnormalities of dystrophin expression. The muscle biopsy of definite carriers can look entirely normal.

Regarding the morphological changes, these include increased variation in fibre size, eosinophilic 'hypercontracted fibres', increase in internal nuclei, and even fibre necrosis and phagocytosis, although the latter are found only when there is florid muscle weakness. In only about 10 per cent of symptom-less carriers is there usually any *obvious* abnormality on routine histology. However, careful quantitation of muscle fibre size, internal nuclei, and histochemical fibre type proportions has been claimed to demonstrate abnormalities in around 70 per cent of carriers. These abnormalities can occasionally be detected even when the SCK level is within the normal range.

Various authors have suggested that in carriers there might be a gradual reduction in the number of affected muscle fibres because of their replacement (from proliferating satellite nuclei) by more normal fibres. This may represent the pathological correlate of the described small decline in SCK levels with increasing age in carriers.

While repeated studies of muscle biopsies on DMD carriers have not been performed, several lines of evidence suggest that 'genetic normalization' (that is, the phenomenon by which the repeated cycles of degeneration and regeneration lead to an increase in the number of dystrophin-competent nuclei because of the fusion of dystrophin-positive satellite cells) may occur in carriers (Fig 11.2).

The first evidence derives from studies performed in the female carriers of the *mdx* mouse and the dystrophic dog. These studies clearly show that the

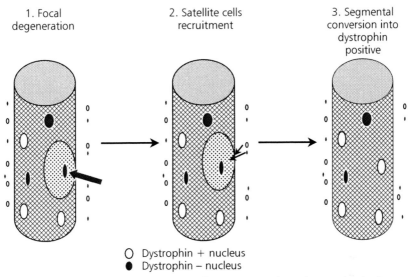

1. Focal degeneration   2. Satellite cells recruitment   3. Segmental conversion into dystrophin positive

○ Dystrophin + nucleus
● Dystrophin − nucleus

Fig. 11.2 The model of biochemical normalization. See colour plate section in the centre of this book.

number of dystrophin-negative fibres declines with age. The pattern of dystrophin expression may also vary depending on the muscle studied. We had the opportunity to study the rectus abdominis of a definite carrier in her sixth decade of life. The rectus abdominis, a non-antigravity muscle that is presumably not significantly affected by dystrophin deficiency (as indicated by the good preservation of its function until late in the course of the disease in DMD), displayed clear clusters of dystrophin-negative and -positive fibres, of roughly equal proportions. In contrast, the quadriceps of the same carrier expressed dystrophin in almost every fibre. We speculate that the stress of the contraction of the antigravity muscle, with its associated degeneration and regeneration, provided the genetic correction in the quadriceps while the rectus abdominis, in which the degeneration and regeneration were absent, still reflected the original random pattern of X-inactivation.

How do we explain, however, the observation that muscle weakness in manifesting carriers tends to get worse, and not improve, over the years? A careful study of DMD carriers by Pegoraro et al. (1995) addresses this complex scenario. These authors studied not only the expression for dystrophin in muscle but also the pattern of X-inactivation in muscle and blood. Their findings suggest two different mechanisms in carriers. One occurs in carriers with a random pattern of X-inactivation; the other in those with a skewed (unfavourable) X-inactivation pattern (Fig 11.2).

In the former group, the phenotype ranged from asymptomatic to mild weakness and the histopathological changes were minor. Interestingly, these patients had higher dystrophin content in muscle than predicted by the number of dystrophin-positive genes. A possibility is that in these patients the relatively low grade of myopathy is not sufficient to trigger a significant recruitment of satellite cells and that the compensation for dystrophin production derives from a 'biochemical' normalization (that is, by the increase of the domain of dystrophin-positive nuclei). On the contrary, patients with skewed X-inactivation showed a more severe phenotype with more significant histopathological changes and were usually classified as 'clinically manifesting carriers'. Pegoraro *et al.* found evidence of 'genetic' normalization in this group of carries, with significantly higher numbers of dystrophin-positive nuclei in muscle compared to leukocytes (in which there is no selective pressure). Unexpectedly, however, in the skewed-inactivated carriers dystrophin was not always produced by genetically dystrophin-positive myonuclei, a production failure possibly due to the unfavourable muscle enviroment. A combination of the 'genetic' and 'biochemical' normalizations probably plays a different role at different ages in differently skewed carriers, therefore explaining not only the diversity of their initial presentation but also of their long-term outcome. From a practical point of view a muscle biopsy is now only very rarely indicated, and only if DNA analysis in the affected DMD patient in the family is not available, for example, in the case of a sister or a maternal aunt of a patient with DMD who died before DNA analysis was available. While DNA screening analysis can detect deletions or duplications, if this is unrevealing there will be the concern that the carrier might be harbouring a mutation not identified by these currently available methods. This occurs in approximately 30 per cent of cases. A muscle biopsy might help to assign the carrier status in this scenario, although its limitations in identifying carriers must be borne in mind.

The consensus would seem to be that convincing and clear-cut muscle dystrophin abnormalities are infrequent in healthy carriers with a normal SCK level. Therefore such studies, which are both invasive and expensive, would seem at least at present to offer little additional information for carrier detection and genetic counselling.

Molecular genetics studies

There have been many attempts to improve the discriminatory value of the SCK test by combining the results with those of other tests, such as muscle pathology and dystrophin expression studies. However, it is now clear that the most useful information is obtained by the direct study of the intragenic mutation, if this is known, or by combining SCK data with information from

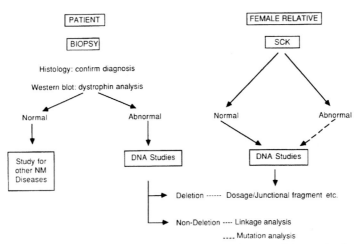

Fig. 11.3 The diagnosis of the affected male and identification of the carrier female in a family with an Xp21 disorder.

linked DNA markers when information on a possible mutation is not available. It is incorrect to consider the value of the SCK test purely in terms of 'detection rate'. It is much preferable to consider the probability (odds) of a woman being a carrier on the basis of not only her SCK level but also pedigree and DNA data. It usually then makes little difference to the final probability estimate in practical terms whether the test result is actually outside the normal range or lies in the upper part of the range.

Finally, the diagnosis of the affected male and the identification of a carrier female in a family has to be seen as an overall problem, data on the former helping to establish the status of the latter (Fig. 11.3).

Calculation of risks

The estimation of genetic risks is usually based on Bayes' theorem. In these calculations four probabilities are considered: prior; conditional; joint; and posterior. The prior probability is based on knowledge of the individual's antecedents and sibs. The conditional probability is the probability of being a carrier or not depending on the individual's SCK level, data from DNA markers, and the number of normal sons she may have had. The product of the prior and conditional probabilities is the joint probability. The final posterior probability of a woman being a carrier is the joint probability of getting the observed information, given she is a carrier, divided by the sum of this probability plus the joint probability of getting the observed information if she is not a carrier. The method of calculation is illustrated in the following examples.

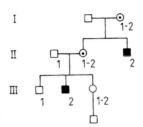

Fig. 11.4 Pedigree of DMD linked to an RFLP, the alleles of which are represented below the pedigree symbols.

Consider the family in Fig. 11.4 where a daughter III$_3$ with a normal son seeks genetic counselling. It would appear that the Duchenne gene and restriction fragment length polymorphism (RFLP) allele-2 are co-inherited in the family. First, we consider the prior probability of III$_3$ being a carrier or not being a carrier which is 0.5. Let us assume that she has an SCK of 40 IU, that she has inherited RFLP allele-2 from her mother, and that the frequency of recombination (θ) between the RFLP and the disease locus is 5 per cent (0.05). Then, if she is a carrier, the (conditional) probability of her having allele-2 is 0.95, that is, 1 minus θ, because crossing-over would not have to occur. Since 56 per cent of controls and 12 per cent of definite carriers have an SCK of 31–50 IU (Table 11.3), the conditional probability of having an SCK of 40 IU if she is a carrier is 0.12.

Finally, the conditional probability of having a normal son if she is a carrier is 0.50. On the other hand if she is not a carrier then these conditional probabilities are, respectively, 0.05 (since crossing-over would now have to occur), 0.56, and 1.00. The calculations are set out as follows.

Probability	Carrier	Not a carrier
Prior	0.50	0.50
Conditional		
Allele-2	0.95	0.05
SCK 40 IU	0.12	0.56
Normal son	0.50	1.00
Joint	0.029	0.014

Her posterior probability of being a carrier is then

$$0.029/(0.029 + 0.014) = 0.674,$$

that is, there is a very high probability (67 per cent) that she is a carrier and therefore any son she has would have a 1 in 3 chance of being affected.

However, suppose she had inherited allele-1 and therefore seemed unlikely to be a carrier (unless crossing-over occurred), yet her SCK level was 100 IU (that is, in the upper part of the normal range). The calculations are then as follows.

Probability	Carrier	Not a carrier
Prior	0.50	0.50
Conditional		
Allele-1	0.05	0.95
SCK 100 IU	0.144	0.015
Normal son	0.50	1.00
Joint	0.002	0.007

Her posterior probability of being a carrier is then

$$0.002/(0.002 + 0.007) = 0.222.$$

Thus, the chance of being a carrier remains high and in this case the probability of a son being affected is roughly 1 in 9.

It should be noted that in these calculations for the sake of simplicity the linkage phase in the mother (whether allele-2 is co-inherited with the Duchenne gene) is assumed and, with a closely linked probe ($\theta < 0.10$), this makes no practical difference to the results. However, nowadays in many families there is only one affected boy. The affected boy in such a family may represent a new mutation and there is also no certainty as to the linkage phase in the family. Let us first consider for the sake of simplicity that in such a family only data on SCK levels are available. Let us assume that a woman who seeks genetic counselling has an SCK of 80 IU, one normal brother, and a sister with an SCK of 60 IU who has an affected son, there being no one else affected in the family. We first have to go back one generation and consider the mother of these two sisters. Like any woman in the population she has a prior probability of being a carrier of 4μ where μ is the mutation rate in both males and females. The reason, put simply, is that the chance of a mutation occurring in either of her maternally or paternally derived X chromosomes is 2μ and the probability that she might have inherited the mutant gene through her mother is also 2μ. We then consider the conditional probabilities, firstly, of her having had a normal son and, secondly, of having had a daughter with an SCK of 60 IU and an affected son. In the case of the daughter we first determine the prior probabilities of her being a carrier or not a carrier given that her mother is or is not a carrier. Secondly, we determine the conditional probabilities of the daughter having an affected son and an SCK level of 60 IU assuming that she is or is not a carrier, and, finally, we determine her joint probabilities. The final overall joint probabilities are arrived at by multiplying the daughter's joint probabilities by her mother's prior probabilities and her mother's conditional probabilities of having a normal son.

The calculations are set out as follows.

Probability	Mother			
	Carrier		**Not a carrier**	
Prior	4μ		$1-4\mu \cong 1$	
Conditional				
A normal son	1/2		1	
Daughter				
	Carrier	Not a carrier	Carrier	Not a carrier
Prior	1/2	1/2	2μ	1
Conditional				
Affected son	1/2	μ	1/2	μ
SCK 60 IU	0.07	0.24	0.07	0.24
Joint (daughter)	0.02	0.12μ	0.07μ	0.24μ
Joint (mother)	0.04μ	$0.24\mu^2$*	0.07μ	0.24μ

* Negligible.

The final posterior probability of the mother being a carrier, taking into account information on her daughter with an affected son, is the sum of the joint probabilities if she is a carrier (columns 1 and 2) divided by the sum of these probabilities plus the sum of the joint probabilities if she is not a carrier (columns 3 and 4), that is,

$$0.04\mu/(0.04\mu + 0.07\mu + 0.24\mu) = 0.11.$$

We now consider the sister who came for counselling who now has a prior probability of being a carrier of 0.055, say 0.06.

Probability	Carrier	Not a carrier
Prior	0.06	0.94
Conditional		
SCK 80 IU	0.16	0.03
Joint	0.010	0.028

Her posterior probability of being a carrier is therefore

$$0.010/(0.010 + 0.028) = 0.26.$$

Thus, despite the fact that both she and her sister have SCK levels within the normal range, the sister who requested counselling still has a high chance (namely, about 1 in 4) of being a carrier.

A general formula for calculating the probability of a woman being a carrier of a *lethal* X-linked disorder that affects either a brother or a son (*there being no one else affected in the family*) has been derived. If h_c and h_m refer respectively to the relative probabilities of normal homozygosity to heterozygosity (Y_1/Y_2 in Table 11.3) in the suspected carrier and her mother, so that, if there is no such information, $h = 1$, and if q is the number of normal brothers and r the number of normal sons, and if s is 1 where a son is affected and 0 if a brother is affected, and t is 0 where a son is affected and 1 if a brother is affected, then the probability (P) of her being a carrier of a *lethal* X-linked disorder is

$$P = (1 + sa)/(1 + sa + ab + tb)$$

where $a = h_m 2^q$ and $b = h_c 2^r$.

It is also helpful to include in these calculations information on SCK levels in all the first-degree postpubertal female relatives of a suspected carrier. Over the years one of us has tested some 1400 potential carriers in over 400 families, in many of which there was only one affected boy. By using Bayesian statistics and combining both pedigree and SCK data, rather than using pedigree data alone, this reduced considerably the proportion of women who fell into the intermediate risk range (Fig. 11.5). Even further separation is possible if DNA data are also included in the calculations.

Finally, even in families with an isolated case of DMD, carrier detection can be improved by using data from a linked RFLP or microsatellite polymorphic marker. The probability of the sister of an affected boy being a carrier (or a subsequent male fetus being affected) depends on whether the individual has the same or a different maternal RFLP (or other markers) from the affected

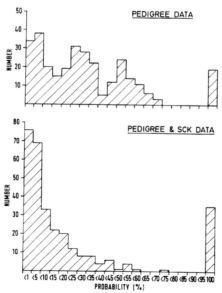

Fig. 11.5 Risks in 300 potential carriers based on: (above) pedigree data alone; (below) pedigree and SCK data combined.

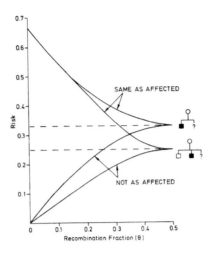

Fig. 11.6 Risks of the sister of an isolated DMD case being a carrier (or a subsequent male fetus being affected), depending on whether the individual has the same or a different maternal RFLP allele from the affected boy.

boy. If the sister has a different allele then, barring crossing-over, she is unlikely to be a carrier. The position is improved the closer the DNA marker is to the disease locus. If θ is, say, 0.05 and she has a different allele from her affected brother, her risk becomes about 1 in 16, or less than 1 in 30 if she also has an unaffected brother (Fig. 11.6). The risks could be reduced even further depending on her actual SCK level.

Information on DNA markers lying on either side of the locus (flanking or bridging markers) and from the maternal grandfather's haplotype is also important and increases the precision. The likelihood that information from a linked RFLP (or other markers) will be helpful (the mother will be heterozygous and the segregation pattern in the family will be informative) increases as the number of alleles at the marker locus increases.

The calculations involved in determining the probability of the mother or sister of an isolated case being a carrier, which takes into account both SCK and RFLP (or other markers) data, are detailed in Emery (1986) and Young (1991). However, they can be somewhat tedious, especially when more than one DNA marker is involved and there are a number of relatives to be considered. All these calculations are now performed using computer programs. Too much reliance on such programs, however, may lead to problems because serious errors can occur if mistakes are inadvertently made in inserting relevant data. When dealing with straightforward familial cases, and in isolated cases where one is only dealing with a single closely linked probe, the calculations can often be performed with a hand calculator.

A guide to the risks of a daughter whose brother is an isolated case being a carrier is given in Table 11.5. The risks depend on her SCK level (the relative probability of normal homozygosity to heterozygosity 'h'), whether she has

Table 11.5 Risks of the sister of an isolated DMD case being a carrier (or of a subsequent male fetus being affected) for different values of h and recombination fraction (θ), and whether the sister (or male fetus) has the same* or a different† RFLP allele from the affected boy. (When $\theta = 0.50$, there are no data on a DNA marker; when $h = 1.0$, there are no data on SCK)

| | Recombination fraction (θ) | | | |
	0.01	0.05	0.10	0.15
$h = 0.1$				
Same:	0.950	0.938	0.923	0.908
Diff:	0.118	0.403	0.577	0.672
$h = 0.2$				
Same:	0.904	0.884	0.858	0.831
Diff:	0.063	0.253	0.405	0.506
$h = 0.5$				
Same:	0.790	0.753	0.707	0.664
Diff:	0.026	0.119	0.214	0.291
$h = 1.0$				
Same:	0.653	0.603	0.547	0.497
Diff:	0.013	0.063	0.120	0.170
$h = 2.0$				
Same:	0.485	0.432	0.376	0.330
Diff:	0.007	0.033	0.064	0.093
$h = 3.0$				
Same:	0.386	0.336	0.287	0.248
Diff:	0.004	0.022	0.043	0.064
$h = 4.0$				
Same:	0.320	0.275	0.232	0.198
Diff:	0.003	0.017	0.033	0.049
$h = 5.0$				
Same:	0.274	0.233	0.194	0.165
Diff:	0.003	0.013	0.027	0.039

$$*\text{Risk} = \left(1+\frac{h(1+4\theta-4\theta^2)}{2-4\theta+4\theta^2}\right)^{-1} \qquad †\text{Risk} = \left(1+\frac{h(3-4\theta+4\theta^2)}{4\theta-4\theta^2}\right)^{-1}$$

the same or a different RFLP (or other markers) allele as her affected brother, and the frequency of recombination (crossing-over) between the RFLP and the disease locus (0.01–0.15). The risks of the mother having another affected son correspond to the entries in the table where $h = 1$ (that is, where in a potential carrier it is assumed there is no information on SCK levels). These risks, however, ignore additional information that might also be available, including the number of normal sons and brothers the mother may have, the mother's SCK level, information from more than one marker, and the haplotype of the maternal grandfather. Nevertheless, the tabulated risks provide at least a first approximation. Note that, until there is more information about subsequent sons and her daughter's status, the risks of the mother being a carrier are *a priori* 2 in 3 and obviously uninfluenced by DNA marker data on her affected son.

One further point is as follows. The carrier status of a female in an *affected family* without a deletion or duplication may be deduced from information obtained at prenatal diagnosis. If a male fetus is found not to have any dystrophin, then clearly the mother must be a carrier (or a germ-line mosaic). If the fetus has normal dystrophin expression then, of course, this tells us nothing of the mother's genotype.

The particular value of linked markers is that they may provide helpful information even in a family where an isolated affected boy is now deceased. Here it may be possible to show, for example, that the male fetus of a sister of the affected boy has inherited the grandpaternal X chromosome haplotype and therefore is unlikely to be affected. Linkage studies may be the only approach to carrier detection when there is not a deletion. It must be remembered that it is important to use a panel of intragenic markers so that the errors due to recombination are reduced. The occurrence of recombination in a family in which it is not known where the mutation lies prevents the staus of an at-risk fetus being unequivocally determined.

Direct carrier detection

Methods of diagnosis that depend on linkage are referred to as indirect since they do not identify the mutation itself but only its location with respect to DNA markers. Methods that aim to identify the mutation are referred to as direct. These latter methods should, at least in theory, make a precise diagnosis possible.

Dosage

This study can be applied to carriers of a dystrophin gene deletion or duplication. Initially, this test was performed by Southern blot analysis with appropriate cDNA probes. A dosage difference between controls and carriers in the ratio 2 : 1 for deletions and 2 : 3 for duplications might be expected. Unfortunately, in most carriers such differences are not convincing. This methodology has been superseded by quantitative polymerase chain reaction (PCR) amplification using fluorescent primers. By using polymorphic markers or exon-specific primers located inside and outside the deleted area, a confident carrier status can be assigned. The technique requires careful standardization, but in experienced hands it is an extremely powerful tool for these studies in carriers.

Junction fragments

A deletion or duplication may generate a so-called 'junction fragment' of altered size if the breakpoint occurs close to a non-deleted exon so that it lies within the restriction fragment detected by a cDNA probe. This is recognized as an additional band on a Southern blot. If a deletion-associated junction fragment occurs in a family, then all affected males and all carrier females in the family will have this additional band. Unfortunately, with Southern blot analysis and cDNA probes, at most only 20 per cent of deletions are associated with an identifiable junction fragment. However, by using field inversion or pulsed-field gel electrophoresis (FIGE, PFGE), the proportion of cases in which a junction fragment is seen can be increased to over 90 per cent. These techniques are technically very demanding, time-consuming, and require expensive equipment. They have been currently almost entirely superseded by the quantitative PCR approach (Fig. 11.7).

RNA studies (PTT test)

A novel approach to carrier detection was developed by Roberts and colleagues in the early 1990s (Roberts *et al.* 1990, 1991). Initially developed for amplifying (by 'nested' PCR) reversely transcribed mRNA from peripheral blood lymphocytes in which dystrophin mRNA is 'illegitimately' transcribed, because of technical difficulties it has more recently been confined to muscle RNA. Amplified RNA is translated into protein using an *in vitro* system and the proteins are

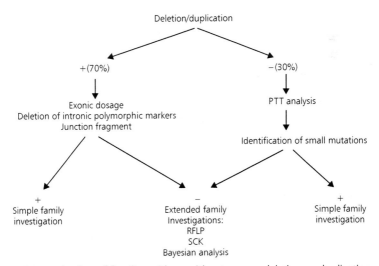

Fig. 11.7 Investigation of families with or without a gene deletion or duplication (unless a point mutation can be detected directly, for example, by a single-strand conformation polymorphism).

run on a gel. If a fragment carries a mutation (out-of-frame deletion or non-sense point mutation, for example), the resulting protein product will be truncated—hence the name of the method, protein truncation test (PTT). The cDNA corresponding to the truncated fragment is than sequenced and the mutation identified.

Automated DNA analysis

Automated methods of analysis are being developed. One of the most recent ones is the DOVAMS (detection of virtually all mutations system), which takes advantage of a modified single-strand polymorphism assay from genomic DNA. The advantage therefore is that it can be performed on ordinary DNA. The technique is, however, still not fully automated. Other approaches that could theoretically be used are automated direct sequencing of the entire dystrophin gene, and the application of DNA microarray technology. Both techniques could theoretically detect the great majority of mutations, but are not available on a large scale.

In conclusion, in familial cases where DNA samples from affected individuals are available and, if a gene deletion or duplication is present, then carrier identification (and prenatal diagnosis) is usually straightforward (Table 11.6). Even when there is only one affected male in the family but DNA is available, then carrier identification is often possible using these methods. A problem arises when the only affected member of the family is now deceased, although with the recent introduction of reliable methods of quantitative PCR it is possible to identify deletions and duplications also in carriers, not only in affected boys. The various approaches available for carrier detection are summarized in Table 11.6.

Prenatal diagnosis

A woman at high risk of having an affected son may choose fetal sexing with selective abortion of any male fetus and in this way be guaranteed a daughter who will not be affected. This is, however, almost invariably not necessary nowadays, as a reliable test for the affected male fetus is possible in most families in which DNA from the propositus is available. Fetal DNA can be extracted using either amniotic fluid cells obtained by transabdominal amniocentesis at about 16–18 weeks of gestation or, more recently, chorion biopsy. Essentially, this latter technique consists of inserting a flexible cannula/catheter either through the cervix or transabdominally into the uterine cavity. Chorionic villi (which are of fetal origin) are carefully removed for DNA, cytogenetic, and other studies (Fig. 11.8). Since this procedure can be performed as early as 10 weeks gestation and the material need not be cultured for DNA or

Table 11.6 Summary of approaches to carrier detection in families with DMD*

Affected male	Available		Unavailable
Deletion/duplication	+	—	
	(70%)	(30%)	
Possible carrier			
SCK	+	+	+
Linkage studies	+	+	(+)
DNA studies			
Dosage	+	—	(+)
Junction fragment	+	—	(+)
In situ hybridization	+	—	(+)
Lymphocyte RNA	+	—	(+)
DNA analysis	+	+	+
Muscle dystrophin	(+)	(+)	(+)

* +, Useful; (+), possible; —, not indicated.

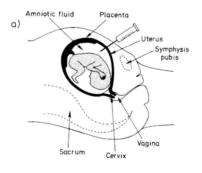

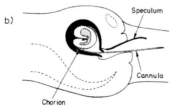

Fig. 11.8 Technique of: (a) transabdominal amniocentesis; (b) chorion biopsy. (From Emery and Malcolm (1995) reprinted with permission of John Wiley and Sons Ltd.)

chromosome studies, a prenatal diagnosis can be made much earlier than with amniocentesis and, if an abortion has to be carried out, it is therefore likely to cause less psychological trauma.

DNA studies on cultured amniotic fluid cells or chorionic biopsy material can establish fetal diagnosis on the basis of linkage studies when there is no deletion or duplication, or by demonstrating a rearrangement at Xp21 in other cases.

Fetal muscle biopsy

Fetal muscle biopsy has also been employed in the past for the diagnosis of an affected fetus. The technique involves inserting a trocar and cannula through the myometrium into the amniotic cavity under ultrasonographic guidance in the second trimester of pregnancy. Diagnosis is then based on histological and dystrophin immunohistochemical studies on the biopsied material, and, remarkably, at birth there is little more than a small scar in the biopsy region. The technique is, however, difficult and the possibility of fetal loss can be high.

Fetal muscle dystrophin

In the normal embryo dystrophin first appears in the sarcolemma at the peripheral ends of the myotubes immediately adjacent to the tendons. In the fetus it appears throughout the entire myofibre, becoming restricted to the sarcolemma only later.

Examination of muscle tissue from fetuses affected with DMD aborted in the second trimester of pregnancy has revealed a complete absence of dystrophin in some fetuses as well as an increased variation in fibre size and an increased number of hypercontracted fibres with increase in intracellular Ca^{2+}, which confirms that these histological changes are, in fact, an early manifestation of the dystrophic process. The possibility of detecting truncated forms of dystrophin in a DMD fetus has also been reported, highlighting the importance of using a panel of antidystrophin antibodies, as discussed in Chapter 4. These immunohistochemical studies could be diagnostically important where no mutation is detectable at the DNA level.

Furthermore, such studies can be very important in helping to establish the carrier status of a mother when DNA is either unavailable from other affected relatives or is uninformative. The demonstration of a significant defect in fetal muscle dystrophin would confirm that a mother at risk is a carrier. In other cases where haplotype information is available in an affected relative, fetal muscle studies may, in conjunction with haplotype data, prove that a mother is not a carrier. This is clearly shown in the evolution over several years in the management of a family in which the only affected male is deceased (Fig. 11.9).

Germ-line mosaicism

Several authors have reported families with intragenic deletions of the Xp21 locus that were transmitted to more than one offspring by women who showed no evidence of the mutation in their own somatic (leukocyte) cells. An example of this is shown in Fig. 11.10. These findings have been attributed to germ-line, germinal, or gonadal mosaicism. That is, individuals who are

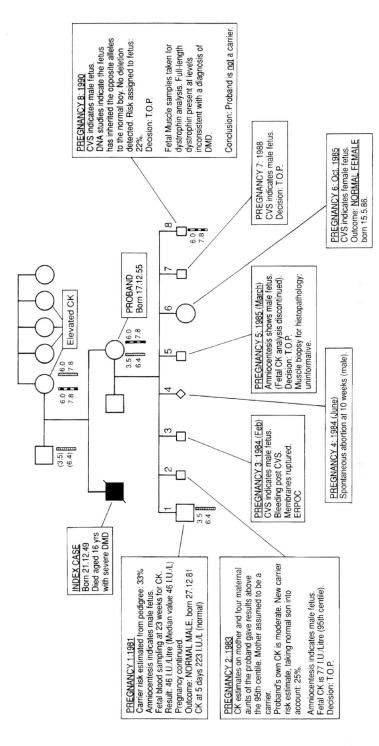

PREGNANCY 8: 1990
CVS indicates male fetus.
DNA studies indicate the fetus
has inherited the opposite alleles
to the normal boy. No deletion
detected. Risk assigned to fetus:
22%.
Decision: T.O.P.

Fetal Muscle samples taken for
dystrophin analysis. Full-length
dystrophin present at levels
inconsistent with a diagnosis of
DMD.

Conclusion: Proband is not a carrier.

PREGNANCY 7: 1988
CVS indicates male fetus.
Decision: T.O.P.

PREGNANCY 6: Oct. 1985
CVS indicates female fetus.
Outcome: NORMAL FEMALE
born 15.5.86.

PREGNANCY 5: 1985 (March)
Amniocentesis shows male fetus.
(Fetal CK analysis discontinued).
Decision: T.O.P.
Muscle biopsy for histopathology:
uninformative.

PREGNANCY 4: 1984 (June)
Spontaneous abortion at 10 weeks (male).

PREGNANCY 3: 1984 (Feb)
CVS indicates male fetus.
Bleeding post CVS.
Membranes ruptured.
ERPOC

PROBAND
Born 17.12.55

Elevated CK

INDEX CASE
Born 21.12.49
Died aged 16 yrs
with severe DMD

PREGNANCY 1: 1981
Carrier risk estimated from pedigree: 33%
Amniocentesis indicates male fetus.
Fetal blood sampling at 23 weeks for CK.
Result: 46 I.U./Litre (Median value 46 I.U./L)
Pregnancy continued
Outcome: NORMAL MALE, born 27.12.81
CK at 5 days 223 I.U./L (normal)

PREGNANCY 2: 1983
CK estimates on mother and four maternal
aunts of the proband gave results above
the 95th centile. Mother assumed to be a
carrier.
Proband's own CK is moderate. New carrier
risk estimate, taking normal son into
account: 25%.

Amniocentesis indicates male fetus.
Fetal CK is 77 I.U./Litre (95th centile).
Decision: T.O.P.

Fig. 11.9 The evolution over several years in the management of a family in which the only affected male was deceased. (Reproduced by kind permission of Drs David E. Barton and Clare Davison.)

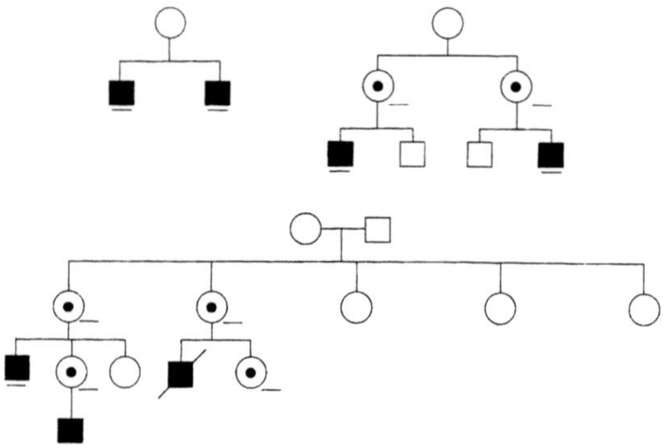

Fig. 11.10 Simplified pedigrees demonstrating germ-line mosaicism in transmitting parents. (—) This indicates a demonstrable Xp21 gene deletion.

phenotypically normal and not genetic carriers nevertheless transmit a mutation to more than one offspring because they harbour a somatic mutation within a fraction of their germ-line cells.

The phenomenon is not restricted to DMD but has also been reported in a variety of other genetic disorders. Though there is as yet no *direct* evidence of germ-line mosaicism in the case of DMD, in dominant lethal osteogenesis imperfecta the causative mutation was detected in one in eight sperm of a normal father who had had two affected infants. In this case the transmitting father's germ-line mosaicism was a reflection of generalized somatic mosaicism. A similar phenomenon was described in a family with DMD in which a transmitting male with mild muscle weakness appears to have been both a somatic and germ-line mosaic.

Estimates of the frequency of germ-line mosaicism among families with DMD have been variously calculated to be between 12 and 20 per cent. Formulae for incorporating germ-line mosaicism into calculations of genetic risk have been proposed. However, from a practical point of view, it means that it can never be assumed that a male fetus born of a mother with a normal genotype will in fact be unaffected. It is therefore advisable to consider prenatal diagnosis in all pregnancies in at least the mother and sisters of an isolated affected boy. In the case of a mother without a deletion who has an affected son, it is important to test with cDNA probes all her daughters to determine if she may be a germ-line mosaic.

Ova transfer and preimplantation diagnosis

The transfer of ova might be indicated in the case of a woman who is at high risk of having an affected son but who for various reasons may not be able to face prenatal diagnosis and abortion. Ova from an unrelated (non-carrier) female may be fertilized *in vitro* by the carrier's husband's sperm. A fertilized ovum is then implanted in the carrier's uterus where it develops normally.

Another possibility is to remove ova by laparoscopy from a carrier female and, having fertilized them with her husband's sperm, allow them to develop *in vitro* until, say, the early blastocyst stage. A single cell is than removed without damaging the conceptus and, by using appropriate DNA technology, it is determined if it will be an affected male. Only unaffected male conceptuses would be reimplanted in the uterus to undergo further development.

An even more intriguing possibility is to remove an ovum and its associated polar body prior to fertilization and, by PCR, amplify the relevant Xp21 sequence in DNA from the polar body. Any X-chromosomal defect detectable in the polar body cannot be present in the ovum, which could then be fertilized *in vitro* and returned to the uterus to undergo further development.

All these techniques are feasible although they are technically very demanding. Few preimplantation diagnoses for DMD have so far been reported.

Summary and conclusions

Since DMD is a serious disorder for which at present there is no effective treatment, much emphasis has been given to prevention. This involves the ascertainment of women likely to have an affected son, and the provision of genetic counselling and prenatal diagnosis for such women. The ascertainment of women at risk could be achieved by screening the entire population for affected boys or by screening women within known affected families. Screening for affected boys in the newborn period has the advantage that such early detection might lead to the prevention of second cases in a family. A number of neonatal screening programmes have been developed with some success.

The major problem in prevention is the detection of female carriers. About 5 to 10 per cent have some degree of muscle involvement but this is rarely serious. A simple test for detecting healthy carriers is the determination of the SCK level. However, today DNA-based techniques are the most reliable means for assigning carrier risk and for prenatal diagnosis. These methods can be divided into indirect methods (linkage analysis) and direct methods that depend upon identifying the mutation itself and include DNA dosage, detection of junction fragments, PTT analysis, and DNA sequencing. Muscle dystrophin studies are only rarely indicated. The extension of DNA studies to the fetus has made prenatal diagnosis possible, either through amniocentesis in the second trimester of pregnancy or, more recently, chorion biopsy in the first trimester of pregnancy. This has also made possible the study of affected fetal muscle, which is providing novel insights into the early stages of the dystrophic process.

Finally, because of the possibility of germ-line mosaicism, it is advisable to consider prenatal diagnosis in all pregnancies in at least the mother and sisters of an isolated affected boy.

References

Emery, A.E.H. and Malcolm, S. (1995). *An introduction to recombinant DNA in Medicine. 2nd edition.* Wiley, Chichester.

Emery, A.E.H. (1986). *Methodology in medical genetics—an introduction to statistical methods,* 2nd edn. Churchill Livingstone, Edinburgh.

Pegoraro, E., Schimke, R.N., and Garcia, C. (1995). Genetic and biochemical normalisation in female carriers of Duchenne muscular dystrophy: evidence for failure of dystrophin production in dystrophin-competent myonuclei. *Neurology* **45**, 677–90.

Roberts, R.G., Bentley, D.R., Barby, T.F.M., Manners, E., and Bobrow, M. (1990). Direct diagnosis of carriers of Duchenne and Becker muscular dystrophy by amplification of lymphocyte RNA. *Lancet* **336**, 1523–6.

Roberts, R.G., Barby, T.F.M., Manners, E., Bobrow, M., and Bentley, D.R. (1991). Direct detection of dystrophin gene rearrangements by analysis of dystrophin mRNA in peripheral blood lymphocytes. *American Journal of Human Genetics* **49**, 298–310.

Schapira, F., Dreyfuss, J.C., Schapira, G., and Démos, J. (1960). Étude de l'aldolase et de la créatine kinase du sérum chez les mères de myopathes. *Revue Française Études Cliniques et Biologiques* **5**, 990–4.

Young, I.D. (1991). *Introduction to risk calculation in genetic counselling.* Oxford University Press, Oxford.

Chapter 12

Genetic counselling

Much emphasis has so far been placed on the probability of a woman being a carrier and the risks of her having an affected son. In genetic counselling these are important issues, but other matters also have to be considered and discussed.

Genetic counselling is essentially a process of communication between the counsellor and those who seek counselling. Information to be communicated falls roughly into two main areas. First, information about the nature of the disorder: its severity and prognosis and whether or not there is any effective therapy, what the genetic mechanism is that caused the disease, and what are the risks of its occurring in relatives. Secondly, information on the available options open to a couple who are found to be at risk of transmitting the disease. The latter may include discussions of contraception, sterilization, prenatal diagnosis, and abortion.

When discussing the disease, the genetic counsellor has to present an accurate picture, even if it is depressing and disturbing, if the parents are to make a reasoned decision about future children. Such discussions require considerable sensitivity and tact when the parents already have a young affected child. It is not uncommon for those involved in both the management of the disease and in counselling to find themselves in the dilemma of having to maintain an optimistic outlook for the affected child while emphasizing the seriousness of the disorder when discussing its possible recurrence in any future children.

Having discussed at length the more medical aspects of the disease, the counsellor then proceeds to explain the genetic mechanism that caused it and the risks of recurrence in terms that are understandable to the individual couple. A preoccupation with risk figures can often be confusing and is best avoided. Often couples merely want to know if there is any chance at all that it could occur again. In many cases genetic mechanisms and recurrence risks need to be discussed only in broad terms. In any event the actual interpretation of risks is very subjective—what might be an acceptable risk to one couple may be quite unacceptable to another. Nevertheless, risks form a useful basis for further discussions and can be a significant factor in influencing decision-making. One important fact that may have to be explained is that, being genetic, the parents cannot hold themselves in any way responsible for the disease, and every effort should be made to dispel feelings of guilt and recrimination that they may be harbouring.

If the risks are considered to be unacceptably high, the options available include family limitation, contraception, prenatal diagnosis, and abortion, and perhaps preimplantation diagnosis and other techniques. Contraception in this context requires expert advice because the results of failure will be far more devastating than when it is practised for purely social and economic reasons. A deep fear of having an affected child may well generate serious psychosexual problems and, for this reason, some definitive form of contraception may well have to be considered, such as tubal ligation or vasectomy. The effects of sterilization when performed on healthy women whose families are complete are likely to be entirely beneficial. But in a young woman in a family with Duchenne muscular dystrophy (DMD) who either has no children or perhaps only the one affected child, it may have significant psychological sequelae. Counselling is especially important in these cases. To some couples sexual abstinence may be the only acceptable alternative.

Prenatal diagnosis has added a whole new dimension to genetic counselling and, when the result is negative, the reassurance it gives is entirely beneficial. But therapeutic abortion can cause considerable psychological trauma in many women and, in those genetic disorders where prenatal diagnosis is possible, after termination of pregnancy following the diagnosis of an affected fetus, a significant proportion of mothers decline to undergo the procedure again. Sensitive counselling is therefore essential both at the time of prenatal diagnosis and during the period following a therapeutic abortion. Although significant psychological trauma may be an unavoidable consequence of selective abortion, the alternative birth of an affected child is usually accompanied by even more intense feelings of guilt and depression.

As a prelude to genetic counselling it is important to divine a couple's educational and social background, their religious attitudes, and, if possible, something of their marital relationship if information is to be presented most effectively and sensitively. The counsellor may sense that for various ethical and other reasons contraception, sterilization, or prenatal diagnosis are unacceptable to a couple. These matters should then not be discussed further. The genetic counsellor's role is to inform and guide but not to coerce or impose his or her own views.

The various factors that influence the reproductive decisions after genetic counselling are complex, variable, and personal.

Non-directive counselling

The genetic counsellor's role, until relatively recently, was often seen purely in medical and scientific terms: to establish a precise genetic diagnosis and to communicate factual information about the disease and its genetics. However, more emphasis is now being given to an appreciation of the psychological aspects of counselling—a change from what Kessler in 1979 referred to as 'content-oriented to person-oriented' counselling. This change has been brought about by several factors. First, a disabling genetic disorder such as DMD often has profound psychological effects on the immediate family. Secondly, these effects may have long-term consequences and frequently extend to other relatives. Thirdly, it has been found that couples sometimes opt for a course of action that may well be at variance with what the counsellor might have regarded as 'reasonable'. For example, in a prospective follow-up study some years ago carried out by one of us, of 200 consecutive couples seen in a genetic counselling clinic with various genetic disorders, a proportion of those told that they were at risk of having an affected child were undeterred and actually planned further pregnancies. At first sight such behaviour might seem irresponsible but on careful questioning in almost all cases the reasons for planning further children were often very understandable when considered from the parents' point of view. In some cases further pregnancies were planned because, after seeing the effects of a disorder in a previous child or in one of the parents, it was not considered sufficiently serious (congenital cataract, congenital deafness, peroneal muscular atrophy), or prenatal diagnosis was available (Sandhoff's disease, X-linked mental retardation). In other cases the parents planned further pregnancies because, if a subsequent child were affected, it would not survive (renal agenesis) or, if it survived, it would succumb within a year or so (Werdnig–Hoffmann disease). There was a small but lamentable group of couples who had no living children and dearly wanted a family at whatever cost.

Thus, a course of action that might seem irresponsible to one person may seem eminently reasonable to another. The choice should be the individual's prerogative, always provided that it is made in the full knowledge of all the facts and possible consequences. Since the genetic counsellor's role is to help couples arrive at decisions that are the best ones for themselves, genetic counselling should never be directive. Nevertheless, because DMD is such a serious and distressing condition, most counsellors may hope that couples at risk will exercise caution.

Timing of counselling—the coping process

For really successful counselling it is essential to recognize the problems of attempting to communicate information of a personal and delicate nature in a situation when the parents may not yet have recovered from the shock of the diagnosis. They may well be harbouring feelings of guilt, recrimination, and lowered self-esteem. They may be angry and tense or just numbed by the situation. But all will be under considerable stress. The psychological sequence of events that follows the initial diagnosis is referred to as the 'coping process' and is similar in other stressful situations such as bereavement. Parents with a child with DMD have to face two major stressful events: at the time the diagnosis is first made; and later when the affected boy dies. On both these occasions the family will require considerable support from all those concerned—paediatricians, physicians, geneticists, genetic associates, social workers, and nurses. It should also be remembered that the father may be just as affected as the mother but, since men often do not express their emotions readily, this may be underestimated or even go unrecognized.

Five sequential stages have been recognized in the coping process (Emery and Pullen 1984):

- shock and denial;
- anxiety;
- anger and guilt;
- depression;
- psychological homeostasis.

The duration of each stage varies from individual to individual. Very rarely, a parent may never progress beyond the stage of denial, while a few may reach the stage of depression and remain at this stage. The genetic counsellor has to recognize the existence of these stages and to tailor his or her counselling accordingly. He/she has to appreciate that the assimilation of information and the process of decision-making will be very much influenced by the stage in the coping process that a parent has reached.

At the very beginning, the parent may be unable to accept that the child is affected, and at this stage sympathy and compassion are required until acceptance occurs. Anxiety impairs judgement and reason, and at this stage the counsellor should provide support and encourage the sharing of emotions. Information may have to be repeated on a number of occasions if it is to be fully understood and appreciated. The most difficult stage for the counsellor is when the parent is angry and resentful. Hostility may well be directed towards the counsellor. This has to be accepted as being part of the coping process and not taken personally. Gentle persuasion is indicated, although sometimes it may be necessary to withdraw temporarily and make arrangements for a later appointment when the parent's hostility and resentment may have been tempered. At the stage of depression the effects may be such as to necessitate some form of antidepressant therapy but it is probably at this stage that genetic counselling can begin more earnestly. Counselling should not be postponed until homeostasis has been reached, although obviously information will be better received and understood and decisions will be more rational at this last stage.

Genetic counselling is part of the general counselling that parents with an affected child are given, and it calls for special knowledge and skills on the part of the counsellor.

Who should be offered genetic counselling?

Geneticists tend to consider risks greater than one in 10 as being 'high' and less than one in 20 as being 'low'. This is based on early studies that tended to show that, in general, couples are more likely to be deterred from planning a pregnancy when the risk is greater than one in 10, but less so if it is less than one in 20. However, it is difficult to extrapolate from responses to genetic disorders in general to one disease in particular, such as DMD, because the so-called 'burden' of a disorder has to be included in the equation. By this is meant the psychological and, to a lesser extent, the social and economic problems attendant on having a child with a serious genetic disorder. In some disorders, such as Werdnig–Hoffman disease, although the burden is great it is of limited duration and therefore possibly more acceptable than in DMD where the affected child survives for many years, becoming progressively incapacitated. There is good evidence that couples are often more influenced by the burden of a disease than by the actual risks of recurrence. Thus, concern among relatives about the disorder occurring in their children is only partly a reflection of their risk. It is also tempered by their individual views of the 'burden' of the disease.

In part for logistical reasons, it has sometimes been suggested that genetic counselling in DMD might be restricted to those women whose *a priori* risk is greater than 1 in 10. But this does not seem entirely justified because affected boys have sometimes been born to mothers whose risk had been estimated to be less than 1 in 20. There would seem every reason to offer counselling where appropriate to all first- and second-degree female relatives of affected boys as well as to any other relative who may be anxious.

Effects of genetic counselling

The effects of genetic counselling and prenatal diagnosis in DMD can be assessed in various ways: in relation to changes in the incidence of the disorder in a community the reproductive behaviour of those counselled; and the social and psychological effects on the family.

The effects on population incidence have already been discussed where it was concluded that at best this could be reduced to the occurrence of new mutations, which in the past represented about one-third of cases.

The effects on the reproductive behaviour of individual women who had been counselled in regards to DMD were assessed in several studies in the 1970s and 1980s. In general, those who were at high risk were often deterred after counselling and either avoided pregnancy altogether, or opted for prenatal diagnosis in any future pregnancy. In Brazil a high proportion of those at low risk were also deterred but this may reflect the use of the information by women to gain priority help from family planning centres.

These follow-up studies also confirmed that the proportion of affected boys among births to mothers considered to be at high risk was, as expected, greater than among mothers considered to be at low risk.

However, all these studies were carried out before accurate carrier detection and prenatal diagnosis became possible using DNA markers. Now that the element of uncertainty has been removed it would be interesting to compare these early findings with studies carried out today to assess the effects of counselling and changes in population incidence of the disorder.

The social and psychological effects of genetic counselling in DMD are much more difficult to assess. A common complaint from parents is that at the time of diagnosis they were experiencing considerable stress, making it difficult to accept information at all. In one extensive study in the UK, Firth (1983) reported the results of interviews with 53 families. In only 18 were both parents told of the diagnosis together. Many of the parents who had been alone when told described how their distress was heightened by having to break the news to their spouse. A third of the parents were not satisfied with the way the information had been conveyed, which was often inadequate and with no follow-up. Although conveying information about a diagnosis is only part of counselling, it is an important part. It is difficult to see how, if at this stage a good rapport has not been established with a couple, any meaningful dialogue can follow later. On the basis of her findings Firth made some recommendations: parents should be told of the diagnosis as soon as possible, together and in private, and a series of contacts should be planned not only with the paediatrician but with other health-care professionals involved with the disease who can provide long-term support for the family. Since her report appeared in 1983 there have been many changes. More help and guidance is now being given to families, but there is always room, for improvement. Some years ago a Working Party of the National Association for Mental Health concluded:

> ... telling the parents is only a first step in the continuing management of the handi-
> capped child. It is not an end in itself and unless it leads correctly on to the appropriate

> involvement of other professional workers it would largely have failed in its primary object of securing for the handicapped child the fullest possible developmental goals and an accepted place in the family. (Carr and Oppé 1971)

Although these sentiments were expressed in regard to handicap in general, they are also relevant to DMD. Establishing the diagnosis and proffering genetic counselling should only be the beginning of the health professionals' involvement with the parents and the affected child. Their continuing support may well be required for several years to come.

A very readable series of reviews of the great variety of psychosocial problems associated with DMD and other neuromuscular disorders is provided by Charash *et al.* (1991). This and Firth's (1983) report should be carefully considered by anyone becoming involved in counselling families with DMD.

Summary and conclusions

Genetic counselling is essentially a process of communication between the counsellor and those who seek counselling. The information to be communicated concerns, firstly, the disease itself, the genetic mechanism that caused it, and the risks of recurrence and, secondly, the options available if the risks are considered unacceptably high. These include contraception, sterilization, prenatal diagnosis, and abortion, each of which may in itself have important psychological sequelae and require counselling. Some couples, for various ethical and other reasons, may be unable to accept these options. This is their prerogative for genetic counselling should not be directive but help couples reach a decision that is the best one for themselves.

It is particularly important to recognize the psychological aspects of genetic counselling and the sequence of events that follows the initial diagnosis and that is referred to as the 'coping process'. This involves five sequential stages: shock and denial; anxiety; anger and guilt; depression; and, finally, psychological homeostasis. Each stage requires counselling to be tailored accordingly for only in this way will it be at all effective and will rational decisions be made.

Concern about the disorder occurring in various relatives is tempered by considerations of the 'burden' of the disease as well as the individual's risks, and counselling should be offered to all those female relatives who are anxious about the problem.

The effects of genetic counselling can be assessed in several ways. There are indications that the population incidence is being reduced to the occurrence of new mutations. Familial cases are now becoming rare. Studies of the reproductive behaviour of individual women who have been counselled indicate that those at high risk are very largely deterred from pregnancy unless coupled with prenatal diagnosis. Finally, the social and psychological effects of genetic counselling can be assessed, but so far this has received little attention in the case of DMD. Indications are that there is often some dissatisfaction with the way in which the diagnosis is first made and lack of subsequent follow-up. There is a real need to ensure that parents are told accurately and compassionately as soon as possible. Thereafter a series of contacts can be offered and planned with various health-care professionals involved with the disease. The latter can then provide, if need be, long-term support for the family as a whole.

References and further reading

Carr, E.F. and Oppé, T.E. (1971). The birth of an abnormal child: telling the parents. *Lancet* ii, 1075–7.

Charash, L.I., Lovelace, R.E., Leach, C.F., Kutscher, A.H., Goldberg, J., and Roye, D.P. Jr (ed.) (1991). *Muscular dystrophy and other neuromuscular diseases: psychosocial issues.* Haworth Press, New York.

Emery, A.E.H. and Pullen, I.M. (ed.) (1984). *Psychological aspects of genetic counselling.* Academic Press, London.

Firth, M.A. (1983). Diagnosis of Duchenne muscular dystrophy: experiences of parents and sufferer. *British Medical Journal* **286**, 700–1.

Harper, P.S. (1988). *Practical genetic counselling*, 5th edition. Butterworth Heinemann.

Kessler, S. (1979). The psychological foundations of genetic counseling. In *Genetic counseling—psychological dimensions* (ed. S. Kessler), pp. 17–33. Academic Press, New York.

Chapter 13

Management

With the identification and charaterization of the defective protein in Duchenne and Becker muscular dystrophies (DMD and BMD, respectively), prospects for a rational therapy at last seemed a reality. However, despite the advances in understanding the molecular basis for DMD and the recent limited success of gene- and cell-therapy-based approaches in the *mdx* mouse, any realistic prospect for an effective curative treatment for DMD still remains elusive. Palliative treatment therefore represents an essential tool to enhance affected boys' quality of life. Recent evidence also suggests that it can prolong life. Palliative treatment includes the prevention of skeletal deformities and appropriate surgical intervention that can improve or stabilize motor function in selected patients. Early detection and treatment of respiratory and cardiac complications has a significant role in reducing morbidity and improving quality of life and survival. Several drug treatments have also been proposed and tried in DMD of which glucocorticoids appear to have the greatest effect. Several detailed reviews on the subject have been written. We refer to two European Neuromuscular Centre (ENMC) workshops for an overview of this topic (Dubowitz 1997; 2000). For a practical and comprehensive guide on how to raise a child with DMD, please refer to Thompson *et al.* (1999).

General management

In the early stages of the disease, and up to the time at which walking becomes difficult, parents should be encouraged to let their son lead as normal a life as possible. Prolonged bed rest for any intercurrent infection should be avoided, particularly after early childhood when it can precipitate loss of ambulation. Similarly, early remobilization following limb fractures is of fundamental importance in this condition. Some of the more important aspects of physical management are summarized in Table 13.1.

Feeding and nutritional aspects

It would seem hardly necessary to emphasize the need to maintain good health in general. There is no evidence that 'megavitamin therapy' is of any value in the disease, and in any event it may have serious side-effects and could

Table 13.1 Physical management in Duchenne muscular dystrophy

Promotion of ambulation
Weight control
Exercise: active/passive
Splints
Tenotomies and orthoses for ambulation
Prevention of deformities
Posture/support/orthoses
Passive exercise/stretching
Surgery
Preservation of respiratory function

actually be harmful. Adequate intake of dietary fibre is important because of frequent problems with constipation, especially evident in the late stages of the disease and often requiring pharmacological intervention. Excess weight gain should be avoided since it will overburden the already compromised musculature. Furthermore, postoperative and nursing care in general is more difficult in obese children. In addition, the propensity of boys with DMD to put on excessive weight is an important factor to take into account when considering the use of glucocorticoids. Families with boys affected by DMD should be given dietary advice and an early consultation with the dietician may be useful. Griffiths and Edwards (1988) have published a chart that allows the determination of the ideal weight for a boy with DMD. In overweight boys, controlled weight reduction by decreased caloric intake is effective and safe. Oral hygiene is also essential.

In the advanced stages of the disease, undernutrition becomes a common problem, with a prevalence of 54 per cent in DMD by the age of 18 years. Weight loss at these stages is secondary to a high incidence of dysphagia, and may be further aggravated by choking episodes, fear of choking, and poor neck posture secondary to scoliosis. Loss of appetite and weight loss in a non-ambulant patient might also be secondary to nocturnal hypoventilation. A full feeding assessment and an overnight sleep O_2 saturation monitoring study is recommended for individuals in the non-ambulant stages of DMD with failure to thrive.

Treatment may involve improving seating posture for meal times, caloric supplementation, and, in very rare instances, gastrostomy feeding. Nasogastric supplementary feeding may sometimes be used as a transient means to recover weight following an acute weight loss, such as that following a prolonged chest infection.

Physical therapies

Active exercise

A question often asked is whether the parents should encourage active exercise in the belief that this might improve muscle strength or perhaps help preserve what strength remains. Early studies of any possible beneficial effects of exercise in DMD are difficult to interpret for various methodological reasons. But it is clear that an overtly aggressive approach to physical activity could well be counterproductive and possibly aggravate the cardiomyopathy that is a concomitant of the disease. Furthermore, the detrimental effect of excessive physical activity is highlighted in the various animal models of muscular dystrophy. In *mdx* mice a regular programme of exercise or activity against resistance accelerates the course of the disease and worsens the pathology. Therefore, exercise against resistance is not recommended in DMD. In any event, activities involving recreational sports are generally more likely to win long-term adherence. Swimming is particularly valuable as the buoyancy of the water makes exercises easier to perform. Cycling can also be beneficial, although quite early on boys with DMD find this difficult. The best advice would be to encourage normal physical activities as far as they are possible.

Passive exercise and physiotherapy

Various studies have shown that passive stretching exercises are valuable in preventing or at least delaying the development of muscle contractures, which are especially likely to develop in the late stages of the ambulation phase or once the child becomes chairbound.

The role of physiotherapy in DMD goes, however, beyond the simple prevention of skeletal deformities. Several detailed physiotherapy assessment protocols have been formulated for comprehensive evaluation of strength and function in DMD and enable accurate monitoring of disease progression, timing of therapeutic interventions, and documentation of the effects of any intervention. These have been reviewed by Manzur (2001). These standardized protocols are also useful for performing multicentre research studies.

There are essentially two main aspects of physiotherapeutic regimens: prevention of deformities and promotion of ambulation. The prevention of deformities is particularly important in the early phases of the disease and includes passive stretching of the Achilles tendon and the knee, hip, shoulder, and, to a lesser extent, elbow and wrist joints. These stretching exercises should be carried out daily in children with DMD and this can be best accomplished by the parents, after an induction session with a professional physiotherapist. Sylvia Hyde (1984) has produced a helpful guide to such exercises for parents to use in the home (Fig. 13.1). A practical list of the exercises indicated at different stages of the disorder is indicated in Table 13.2. The emphasis is on firmness and kindness and the aim is to prevent contractures developing. There is no doubt that a routine of passive exercises each day, perhaps after a nightly bath, will help prevent contractures. Despite being demanding and time-consuming,

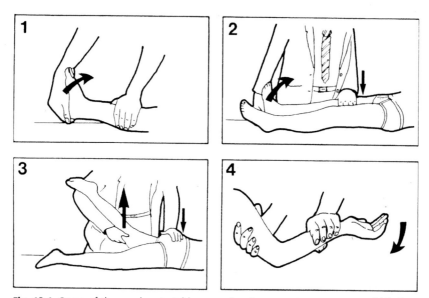

Fig. 13.1 Some of the passive stretching exercises to prevent contractures of (1) the tendo Achilles and (2) the knee, (3) the hip, and (4) the elbow joints. (After Hyde (1984) with permission.)

Table 13.2 Practical approach to prevention of deformities in the ambulant stages of DMD

Intervention*	Timing	Comment
TA stretching	As soon as contractures are present	Typically already at diagnosis
Night splints	If loss ≥ 20°	Commonly a few years after diagnosis
Hip stretching	When contractures detected	Common towards late phasesof ambulation
ITB stretching	When contractures detected	May occur during late phases of ambulation
Knee stretching	When contractures detected	Rarely needed; may be found inchildren with asymmetrical ankle contractures

* TA, Achilles tendon; ITB, ileotibial band.

it offers one of the few opportunities where parents can feel involved in doing something for their son.

Night splints are invaluable aids to the prevention of tightness of the Achilles tendons. They should always be prescribed once the ankles cannot be dorsiflexed beyond the neutral position. While the use of long-leg night splints in order to help prevent the development of contractures of the ankle and knee joints is theoretically more beneficial than using isolated ankle splints, many children find long-leg splints uncomfortable and, in our experience, compliance is very low. The use of ankle splints is well tolerated by most children, especially if their use is introduced gradually over a period of a week while the child is asleep.

In a prospective study of passive stretching and splintage in boys with DMD, a delay in loss of dorsiflexion was noted in the boys whose families complied with treatment. In the boys who were non-compliant, the deterioration in functional level was most marked. The effectiveness of night splints (ankle–foot orthoses) has been demonstrated in a randomized study in ambulant boys with DMD. The best results were obtained in those children who, in addition to the stretching, also had the night splints (Hyde *et al.* 2000). While it has not been formally proven in randomized studies that these measures will prolong ambulation, it is clear from various open studies that early institution of physiotherapy helps in prolongation of ambulation.

We currently encourage children with DMD to wear ankle night splints whenever a significant (that is more than 20 degrees) limited dorsiflexion has occurred (Table 13.2). In our practice the rate of compliance is very high (more than 90 per cent).

Early surgery

In some centres Achilles tenotomy is proposed in the *early* stages of the disease. The procedure, namely, the *early* release of contractures in ambulant boys with percutaneous tendo Achilles lengthening, hip and knee flexion contracture release, and bilateral dissection of tensor fascia lata, was proposed by Rideau in 1986 (Rideau *et al.* 1986). It was claimed that this surgery improved gait and reduced Gowers' time. However, controlled trials of *early* release of lower limb contractures following the protocol introduced by Rideau have failed to show any benefit. *Early* release of lower limb contractures in DMD as a routine treatment cannot therefore be currently recommended.

Prolongation of walking with orthoses

Prolongation of walking in DMD can be achieved by fitting light plastic or polypropylene long-leg fitted orthoses with an ischial supporting lip at the time of increasing difficulty in walking. This approach to management was first introduced by Vignos and Siegel in the 1960s (Spencer and Vignos 1962; Vignos *et al.* 1963; Siegel *et al.* 1968). Their rehabilitation programme of Achilles tenotomy and provision of knee–ankle–foot orthoses (KAFOs) resulted in an average prolongation of walking of 2 years in boys with DMD. If an equino-varus deformity is already present, and this is almost the rule after loss of ambulation, an Achilles tenotomy may be necessary in order to fit the orthoses. This should be performed percutaneously. Compared to the surgical elonga-tion of the Achilles tendon this technique has the advantage of being rapid and not very painful. In our experience almost all boys requiring ischial-bearing orthoses will have sufficient Achilles tendon contractures requiring surgical intervention to fit the orthoses. Some not requiring tenotomy at first and walking regularly in their orthoses may subsequently have problems with Achilles tendon tightening and require a tenotomy later.

A small proportion of children requiring ischial-bearing orthoses will also have significant hip flexion or ileo-tibial-band contractures. Additional teno-tomy of the hip flexors or tensor fascia lata might be required in these children. This can be combined with Achilles tenotomy in the one operation. However, in our experience multiple level surgery makes rehabilitation more difficult because of the increased pain and the decreased stability. We consider it to be necessary only when major contractures that prevent walking in KAFOs are present. In our clinical practice only 5 per cent of children have required ileo-tibial-band release and less than 1 per cent have required the combination of Achilles tendon, hip flexors, and ileo-tibial-band releases.

The benefits of rehabilitation procedures are that they result in prolongation of walking in orthoses of around 18 months, psychological benefits, and delay in development of progressive scoliosis (Rodillo *et al.* 1988). In our experience KAFOs are constructed of individually moulded polypropylene and aluminium alloy and have the advantage of being strong, light-weight, and unobtrusive as they are worn under the trousers (Fig. 13.2). The orthoses are made the week before surgery and are available when the child is admitted for surgery. The child undergoes surgical intervention at the beginning of the week, with surgery last-ing less than half an hour. The child is fitted in theatre with his night splints. The day after surgery the child has two sessions of standing in his KAFOs, and this is progressively increased during the rest of the week . Usually, by the end of the first week or the middle of the second, children are able to walk independently.

The mean for prolongation of independent walking from various published studies is approximately 24 months. Often children will continue to be able to stand in KAFOs, often with the help of a standing frame, for a further 18–24 months after the loss of the ability to walk with KAFOs.

Because of the unpredictable course of the disease, especially shortly before the loss of independent ambulation, and the narrow window of opportunity

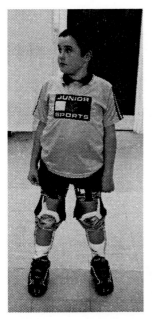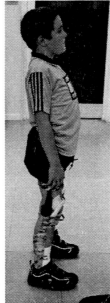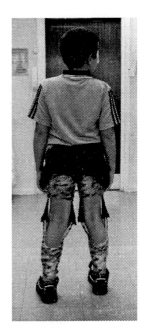

Fig. 13.2 A standing child in KAFOs.

in which to successfully rehabilitate children in KAFOs, it is vital to review boys with DMD regularly at a centre where facilities for rehabilitation are available. The advantages include psychological preparation of the family for loss of walking, informing them about the option of rehabilitation in callipers, and choosing the appropriate timing of intervention.

In our experience the application of orthoses does not accelerate deterioration in muscle power and, in fact, there may be a slight increase for a time.

Late surgery

Late surgery to correct severe equinovarus deformities in the non-ambulant phase of the disease might be required if pressure sores develop. Occasionally, surgery may be requested for cosmetic reasons in children who wish to maintain their feet in a satisfactory position and wear ordinary shoes.

Standing frames and walkers

These are devices that allow a boy who can no longer stand unaided to achieve and maintain an upright position (Fig. 13.3). The advantage of this equipment is that it allows the maintenance of an upright position and provides stretching of the leg joints, in addition to the psychological benefits of standing.

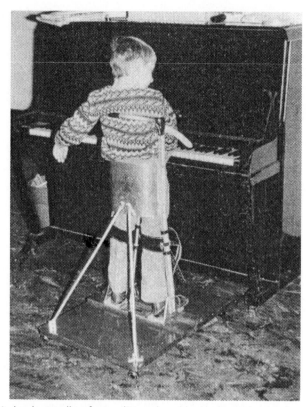

Fig. 13.3 A simple standing frame. (Reproduced by kind permission of Dr G.M. Cochrane and the Mary Marlborough Lodge.)

However, these aids in general have limited manoeuvrability and may be difficult to introduce into the daily routine unless a dedicated physiotherapist is available for help. As mentioned above, they can be used in combination with KAFOs in the later stage of standing. Modified wheelchairs have also been designed for the same purpose and have the advantage of being directly controlled by the child. However, they are much more expensive than ordinary wheelchairs.

An extension of the standing frame is the swivel walker whereby the patient, while being maintained in an upright position, can progress forward by swinging forward the hips. The main problem in DMD is hip and truncal weakness, so that their use is limited compared to other orthoses such as KAFOs. Considering their cost and the limited functional benefit in children with DMD, they are very rarely used.

Surgery for scoliosis

Once an affected boy has lost the ability to walk, joint contractures and scoliosis soon develop. Although contractures are not a serious problem, their development does limit whatever limb movement remains and can also make dressing and lying in bed difficult. Scoliosis, on the other hand, is a serious complication. Sitting becomes difficult and uncomfortable but, more importantly, progressive thoracic deformity restricts adequate pulmonary ventilation and aggravates respiratory problems resulting from weakness of the intercostal muscles. Respiratory impairment becomes a major threat to life and increases once the child is chairbound (Fig. 13.4). It should be noted, however, that not all boys develop scoliosis. A small proportion develop hyperlordosis and some retain more or less a normal spinal curvature. Only exceptionally is spinal curvature evident before loss of ambulation.

There are several ways in which the development of scoliosis can be limited or delayed. The most important one is the prolongation of ambulation, followed by the adoption of a correct sitting posture and the fitting of an orthosis.

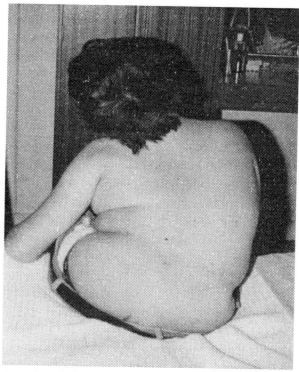

Fig. 13.4 Untreated scoliosis.

From early on, even before ambulation is lost, it is important to emphasize a habit of adopting a correct sitting position. Once confined to a wheelchair this becomes especially important. A firm back support and special seating (for example, the Toronto seat) including a thoracic support if needed will help, but such measures on their own are likely to have only a limited effect. Individually designed body jackets or braces (Figs 13.5 and 13.6), fitted when a boy first becomes confined to a wheelchair and before the onset of a significant scoliosis, may be more helpful. Such measures, however, can only slow down the progression of scoliosis and are neither comfortable nor practical anyway once the severity of curvature has progressed beyond about 50–60 degrees. They have very limited efficacy in obese children. We currently recommend the use of individually casted, low-weight thoracolumbar orthoses in DMD children with a curvature greater than 30 degrees. The brace has to be worn all day while sitting. It should be removed when lying down and when standing or if the child stands with callipers or a standing frame. All children with a curvature of the spine are also assessed by an orthopaedic surgeon as, ultimately, the best solution in order to avoid a severe scoliosis is to resort to surgery.

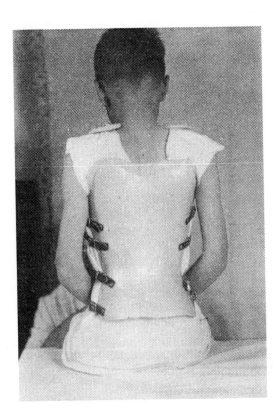

Fig. 13.5 Moulded and fitted back support.

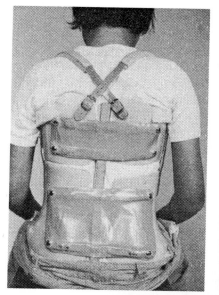
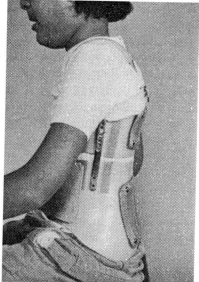
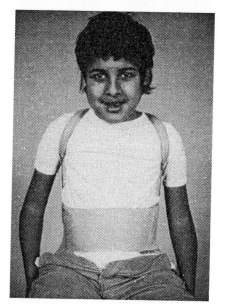

Fig. 13.6 Fitted spinal brace. (Reproduced by kind permission of Dr G.M. Cochrane and the Mary Marlborough Lodge.)

Surgical correction of scoliosis using Harrington rods has now been superseded by the Luque operation in which internal fixation is achieved by each vertebra being individually wired to two stainless steel rods. The rigid stabilization obtained with this technique eliminates the need for postoperative

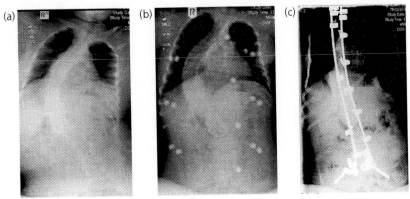

Fig. 13.7 Patient with (a) a severe scoliosis, (b) only partially corrected with a thoracocolumbar brace. (c) Same patient showing good correction following scoliosis surgery using Universal Scoliosis System instrumentation. (Courtesy of Mr. Ian Lefkoski.)

immobilization and therefore reduces the loss of strength and function that follows such immobilization. (Fig. 13.7). While some have recommended the operation as a prophylactic measure before the development of scoliosis, most centres now offer the operation only when scoliosis is more than 30 degrees and has shown an unequivocal tendency to deteriorate.

Spinal surgery is a major procedure that, in addition to the general complication of surgery, is almost invariably associated with a substantial blood loss. This phenomenon is more severe in DMD than in other neuromuscular diseases and it has been speculated that it might be related to smooth muscle involvement in the disease (see Chapter 10, p. 95). In addition, the surgery results in an immediate mild loss of respiratory capacity, although this is counterbalanced by the loss of progressive reduction of respiratory function secondary to the scoliosis. One study some years ago suggested that spinal stabilization in DMD might favourably affect long-term survival. However, more recent studies have now cast doubt on this.

Because of the resultant spinal rigidity and limited spinal movement, boys treated in this way often have to acquire new 'trick' movements for everyday living, and need more frequent turning in bed at night. Boys with stable spines as a result of surgery can be confident that spinal deformity will not increase and often have an enhanced quality of life during the teenage period. The only, but not infrequent, complication of spinal surgery is the development of extension contractures of the neck with progressive neck extension.

In the last two decades the policy at the Hammersmith Hospital has been to consider spinal surgery only in those children who have a definitely progressive scoliosis, with Cobb angles of 30 degrees or more at the beginning of the pubertal growth spurt. In view of the progressive loss of respiratory function characteristic of children with DMD, and of the need to intervene before the forced vital capacity falls below 25 per cent of the predicted value, we carefully monitor all at-risk children every 4–6 months, until they receive spinal surgery or have stopped growing. In our experience patients with curvatures of less than 60 degrees once the spine is fused can be managed conservatively and remain essentially stable. Their overall sitting comfort is not significantly affected by such a curvature. More severe curvatures, however, have a tendency to progressively deteriorate even after the postpubertal bone fusion has occurred. It is important therefore to identify such cases and offer surgical correction.

Surgical–anaesthetic risks

Many children with DMD tolerate surgery and general anaesthesia well, but there are recognized dangers. During anaesthesia, sinus tachycardia, atrial and ventricular fibrillation, and cardiac arrest may occur, even in very young boys aged 3–5 in whom there is no evidence preoperatively of cardiomyopathy or even before the diagnosis of DMD has actually been made.

Postoperatively, other complications may occur, including gastric dilatation and myoglobinuria (rhabdomyolysis). While spontaneous myoglobinuria only very rarely occurs in DMD, it is frequently found postoperatively, and reflects enhanced muscle breakdown. Some patients with myoglobinuria postoperatively have been noted subsequently to be somewhat weaker. The most serious complication of the acute general anaesthetic-induced rhabdomyolysis is hyperpotassaemia followed by cardiac arrest. Unfortunately, this form of rhabdomyolysis does not appear to respond to dantrolene administration. Another important danger with acute rhabdomyolysis and myoglobinuria is the possible development of renal impairment and even acute renal failure postoperatively.

The myoglobinuria (and myoglobinaemia) is probably a direct effect of the anaesthetic agents. Succinylcholine is known to occasionally cause myoglobinuria in normal children, and the apparent increased incidence of myoglobinuria in DMD postoperatively is probably related to the pathophysiology of the disease. Unfortunately, there do not appear to be any factors that preoperatively identify patients likely to develop anaesthesia-related problems. Certainly succinylcholine should be avoided and some other non-depolarizing neuromuscular blocking agent used instead. Interestingly, the risk for rhabdomyolysis appears to be higher in younger children with DMD, perhaps as a result of the better preserved muscle bulk early in life. This complication has also been occasionally reported in manifesting carriers of the disorder undergoing surgery.

Most authors now believe that there is no significant risk of malignant hyperthermia in DMD, and that the rhabdomyolysis and myoglobinuria following general anaesthesia represents a separate phenomenon.

Respiratory problems are also likely postoperatively, especially in boys whose respiratory function is already reduced. Retention of bronchial secretions, resulting from weakness of the respiratory muscles, and the associated weak cough may lead to pneumonitis. Drugs likely to exaggerate respiratory depression, such as barbiturates, have therefore to be used with caution, and postoperative respiratory care and appropriate physiotherapy are essential.

Most of the operative and postoperative problems described in DMD have been based on case reports and are therefore somewhat selective. In the majority of patients there are no serious anaesthetic problems. It is, however, important that the surgeon and anaesthetist appreciate the problems that can occur and be adequately prepared to deal with them should they arise.

Fractures

Fractures occur not infrequently, usually as a result of falls sustained while the boy is still walking but unsteadily, or due to various accidents later on in the course of the disease when the long bones undergo osteoporosis as a result of disuse. In a survey of the prevalence, circumstances, and outcome of fractures in DMD children followed in four UK neuromuscular clinics, around 20 per cent of the 378 patients studied had experienced fractures. Of these, approximately 40 per cent of fractures were in boys aged 8–11 years. Falling was the most common cause. Upper limb fractures were most common in boys using KAFOs, while lower limb fractures predominated in the remaining boys. Twenty per cent of ambulant boys and 27 per cent of those using orthoses permanently lost mobility as a result of the fracture. The fractures themselves, however, heal normally without complications.

Respiratory problems

Impaired pulmonary function is the major factor in morbidity and mortality in DMD. Over 90 per cent of deaths result from pulmonary infection and respiratory failure. Preservation of respiratory function and adequate treatment of respiratory infections are therefore essential elements of patient management.

At the simplest level parents and relatives should be dissuaded from smoking in the rooms used by the affected boy. Vaccination against influenza virus and pneumococcus at the beginning of the winter months is usually recommended in wheelchair-dependent children. Well-designed respiratory exercises are valuable in helping to maintain good pulmonary function. However, these measures alone will not prevent the progressive decrease in pulmonary function. Prophylactic antibiotics are not usually recommended for the prevention of respiratory infections.

Regular pulmonary function tests, the simplest being the assessment of vital capacity using a spirometer, are helpful in monitoring the development of significant impairment even before problems arise, and can be a good prognostic indicator. Significant deterioration begins around the time the boy becomes confined to a wheelchair, and measures of pulmonary function (vital capacity, maximum inspiratory and expiratory pressures), instead of increasing with age as they do normally, remain more or less the same for some time and then in the later stages significantly decrease. Differences between predicted and observed values therefore become more marked as the disease progresses. However, only in the very late stages does actual respiratory failure occur with changes in blood gases.

Attempts to impede the development of scoliosis have already been discussed and certainly have a beneficial effect on respiratory function. Parents can also be instructed in breathing exercises, postural drainage, percussion, and even pharyngeal suction. Some have advocated a 10 minute programme of breathing exercises as part of the daily routine, but respiratory muscle training *per se* seems to have little effect on respiratory function.

Any chest infection must be treated vigorously with antibiotics and physiotherapy. If there is any suggestion that respiratory function is already impaired, then hospitalization is indicated. Practical considerations in the respiratory care of these patients have been reviewed in considerable detail by Smith and colleagues (1987) who provide an extensive and helpful bibliography on the subject.

Assisted ventilation

Impaired respiratory function is the main cause of death in DMD, accounting for approximately 90 per cent of all deaths. Respiratory failure may be sudden, often precipitated by a respiratory infection in a boy whose pulmonary function is already impaired. This poses two questions. Firstly, how can such impairment be detected before serious problems arise? Secondly, what can be done to alleviate this impairment?

Once a boy has become chairbound there is a strong argument for periodically reviewing his condition. Since respiratory insufficiency is first reflected in nocturnal hypoxia and hypercapnoea, suggestive symptoms of this should be specifically sought for since they may be overlooked. These include restless sleep, nightmares, morning confusion, headache, and hypersomnolence during the day. Often appetite is decreased and affected individuals fail to thrive.

Later, clear signs of impaired pulmonary function become evident, including breathlessness and difficulty with speaking. Sleep hypoventilation can be confirmed by overnight oximetry. In clinical practice we recommend regular (yearly) overnight oxygen saturation studies when forced vital capacity (FVC) falls below 40 per cent of normal. However, the nocturnal oxygen saturation is almost invariably normal until the FVC falls below 30 per cent. When this occurs, oxygen saturation studies should be carried out every 6 months and the parents, the children themselves, and other colleagues involved in the care of these patients should be told of the symptoms of nocturnal hypoventilation and its effects. The use of drugs such as protriptyline or theophilline to reduce sleep hypoxia has been extensively studied but they are not helpful.

The most effective way of alleviating impaired respiratory function is assisted ventilation using some form of portable ventilator. This involves intermittent positive pressure with a nasal tube, mouth adaptor, or facial mask. The use of a body shell or cuirass, popular in the 1980s, has now declined. The nasal tube or the facial mask is well tolerated by the great majority of patients. It is important to choose the right moment for starting nocturnal ventilation. In particular, it is important to start the treatment not only when respiratory function is impaired but also when abnormal blood gases are documented in these children. A study performed in France on the use of 'prophylactic' nocturnal ventilation in DMD children not in respiratory failure failed to show any benefit, and was actually detrimental. It is therefore important not only to carefully document the clinical symptoms of respiratory failure but also to document abnormal nocturnal oxygen saturation. If early morning pCO_2 is abnormal, and if day time pCO_2 is also abnormal, then there is strong indication for starting nocturnal ventilation as soon as possible. It has been shown that mean survival once daytime hypercapnoea develops is only 9.7 months without respiratory assistance. Whether nocturnal ventilation should be started in individuals with only nocturnal (*but not diurnal*) hypercapnoea is still controversial and is being investigated.

One of the initial concerns when starting children on nocturnal non-invasive ventilation was related to the assumption that this treatment, initially only offered at night, would inevitably be less effective due to progressive deterioration in respiratory function. This could result in the need for longer periods of ventilation and eventually, after a few years, to 24-hour ventilation. In this instance the use of a tracheostomy was considered a valid alternative but this raised problems related to maintenance and nursing care. More recently, however, various studies have shown that the use of nocturnal non-invasive ventilatory support in DMD is followed by a long period of stabilization. A study on the effects of nasal intermittent positive pressure ventilation (NIPPV) on survival in symptomatic DMD patients with established respiratory failure provides a clear example of this. Nocturnal NIPPV was applied in 23 consecutive DMD patients with ages ranging from 14 to 26 years who presented with diurnal hypercapnia. One- and five-year survival rates were 85 and 73 per cent, respectively. Interestingly, improvements of arterial blood gas tensions were maintained over 5 years with only one case requiring ventilation during the day. Various measures of quality of life were studied and found to be equivalent to those of other groups with non-progressive disorders using the same ventilatory support (Simonds *et al.* 1998). More recently, mouthpiece ventilation has been introduced as an additional respiratory tool for those cases also requiring NIPPV during the day. The combination of nocturnal mask ventilation and the use during the day, if required, of mask or mouth-piece ventilation has resulted in very few if any patients requiring tracheostomy. The mean age of survival of ventilated DMD patients has been evaluated by the group of Bushby from the Newcastle Neuromuscular Centre. They reported that, while the mean age of death in the 1980s before ventilation was introduced was around 19 years of age, this is currently 24.3 years of age, with no patients requiring tracheostomy (Eagle *et al.* 2002). These figures do not take into account the small proportion of patients who develop an early and severe cardiomyopathy, who usually die in cardiac failure before ventilation is started.

Cardiac problems

Conduction system disease occurs very rarely in DMD patients and only a very small proportion die suddenly as a consequence of this complication.

Despite the almost universal cardiac involvement in DMD by the late teens (as demonstrated by electrocardiographic and echocardiographic studies that show left ventricular hypokinesia and enlargement), only rarely do patients develop cardiac symptoms, probably because of the relatively modest load on the heart as a result of the immobility. Hypoventilation and hypoxia can also worsen an already compromised left ventricular function.

Approximately 10–15 per cent of DMD patients might eventually die as a result of the left ventricular failure. In clinically symptomatic patients or in patients with a significant cardiac dysfunction as detected by echocardiography, the use of angiotensin-converting enzyme (ACE) inhibitors, low doses of β blockers, and diuretics, such as frusemide and spironolactone, is currently suggested. While a controlled study of the value of this therapeutic approach has never been performed in DMD, its efficacy in other forms of dilated cardiomyopathy is well recognized, and it would therefore seem sensible to use it also for Duchenne cardiomyopathy.

Table 13.3 Drugs commonly used in DMD cardiomyopathy

Problem	Drug suggested	Comment
Mild left ventricular hypokinesia and dilatation	ACE inhibitor*	Small doses of β blockers are suggested in some protocols
If evidence of cardiac failure	Add diuretics	Usually frusemide or spironolactone
If prominent arrythmias	KCl	Consider defibrillator
If atrial fibrillation	Digoxin and anticoagulant	

* ACE, Angiotensin-converting enzyme.

Long-term prophylactic treatment with cardiac glycosides (digitoxin), although once advocated, has since been shown to have no therapeutic value and is currently not recommended. Verapamil is often used to control a variety of arrhythmias in otherwise normal individuals but is contraindicated in DMD because it may precipitate respiratory failure and heart block. A list of the drugs commonly used in DMD is indicated in Table 13.3.

Psychological problems

Most boys give every impression of being well adapted and of having come to terms with their disability. In fact one expert has said:

> ... it is worthwhile to emphasise that the Duchenne muscular dystrophy patient, after some initial frustration, is really not suffering, has above all no pain, and is on the contrary often quite content or at least acceptingly resigned after he becomes wheelchair-bound. (Zellweger 1975)

It would, however, be entirely wrong to assume that affected boys are emotionally and psychologically unscathed by their disease. Various authors have concluded that emotional problems do occur and that, not unexpectedly, affected boys tend to be more introverted than normal children. In-depth assessment, however, may require some very careful and direct questioning in order to elicit feelings on matters such as isolation, dependency, lack of privacy, and sexual needs.

The emotional reaction of a boy to his disease varies from individual to individual and from family to family. Paramount may be a feeling of isolation because of physical disability—this is more common in children with preserved cognitive function. Recognition that his peers are physically superior may well lead to withdrawal and depression. As the disease advances his dependency on others, and lack of personal privacy, will cause more stress. A proportion may feel physically unattractive. Although some apparently deny that their inability to find sexual satisfaction is a cause of distress, others no doubt do feel this, particularly because their physical disability may preclude any relief they might obtain from masturbation. Later, they have to face the imminence of premature death. While some authors state that many DMD patients accept the concept of premature death without disquiet, others have reported that a major depressive disorder or serious behavioural problems can occur as a reaction to their illness. The more emotionally disturbed tend to come from families with marked conflicts and the behaviour of the parents and normal sibs will influence that of the affected boy. The problems are made worse if the child is ill-informed about the disease. He is more likely to be emotionally stable and better adapted to his problems if the home environment is stable, there is marital harmony, the parents are perceived as being close to each other, and there are open and frequent discussions about his problems with a frank expression of feelings. All too often there is little communication within families about the disorder.

The parents also have to face a great many problems and, again, frank discussions between themselves as well as with health professionals can only be beneficial. Quite apart from the emotional problems associated with coping, there are others of a more social nature that will also produce psychological reactions. Physical handicap, especially when associated with mental handicap, may be viewed as a social stigma and source of embarrassment. As the physical incapacity increases, there will be a restriction on the family's freedom and activities. The parents might find little time or opportunity to be together or to have a holiday. The husband may feel neglected or rejected because of the mother's necessary involvement with their affected son. Coupled with the fear of having another affected child, serious psychosexual problems may arise. In one survey of families, over half had serious marital problems and a quarter had become divorced. On the other hand, in some families the affected child has the effect of actually bringing the parents closer together.

Finally, unaffected sibs are not excluded from the emotional problems that may arise within the family. Overprotection and pampering of an affected boy may result in jealousy and resentment among sibs. Older sisters may adopt a maternal or protective role, yet at the same time harbour increasing concern about their possibly having an affected son.

Emery and Pullen (1984) recognize seven stages in the evolution of a genetic disease within a family, each being associated with different emotional and psychological responses in different members of the family:

1 positive family history;
2 abnormality noticed by parents;

3   abnormality confirmed by family practitioner;

4   diagnosis first made/coping process begins;

5   resolution/adaptation;

6   chronic handicap/progression;

7   death/grieving.

At stage 1 (when there is a family history of DMD), those who see themselves as being at risk of having an affected son are likely to be anxious and concerned. With new improved methods of carrier detection reassurance is often now possible. Otherwise the medical and genetic aspects of the problem will need to be discussed in detail, perhaps on several occasions, until an acceptable course of action is reached. All too often there is a considerable delay between the time when the parents first notice that something appears to be wrong with their son and the time when this is agreed by the family practitioner and the diagnosis is established. Most couples interviewed find this period of uncertainty one of the most trying and unsettling. Unfortunately, current evidence suggests that there is no increased awareness by family practitioners and paediatricians of the possibility of muscular dystrophy. The age at diagnosis of DMD has not changed significantly in the last decade. Stage 4 involves the emotional reaction to the diagnosis and the beginning of the coping process. Stages 5 and 6 involve the reactions of the patient and his parents and sibs to the disease. Parents must be encouraged to take time off and have regular times set aside for themselves. Organizations, such as the Muscular Dystrophy Campaign in Britain, through local set-ups, can provide support and advice and help to reduce feelings of isolation. Open and frank discussions between all members of the family should be encouraged, including the affected boy himself. As Pullen, a psychiatrist experienced in this field, has stated:

> . . . The physically handicapped child must be allowed to talk about his frustrations, disappointments, depression and anxieties for the future. Many people, including parents, do not allow the child to talk about these areas for fear of putting ideas into his head. The ideas certainly are there already but most children are denied the opportunity of communicating them to others. This may make them feel more isolated and abnormal because it prevents others from empathizing accurately with their position. (Emery and Pullen 1984, p. 122)

About a third of parents we have interviewed had great difficulty in talking to each other about the disease.

Finally, at stage 7 parents again should be encouraged to talk honestly about their emotional reactions: their distress, despair, and perhaps anger. The problems of bereavement in muscular dystrophy have been analysed in detail by several authors. Ideally, counselling should not end with the death of the patient but should be available to close relatives until grieving has passed. It is doubtful if the sense of loss and the attendant grief will ever completely pass away. With time, however, there is often a sense of relief after all the years of anxiety and concern. This is natural and not a reason for feeling guilty.

Following these considerations the question arises as to the best way to provide an appropriate psychological and emotional support to the DMD patient and, in particular, if and when psychological support should be offered to the family. Of key importance in this is the attitude and empathy of the staff (medical, nursing, family care officers, and physiotherapy) involved in the care of these patients. A multidisciplinary approach is also very important, as often one colleague might sense or realize a particular problem not necessarily evident to others.

What we suggest in clinical practice is an early and precise diagnosis. The communication of the diagnosis should be performed by a senior physician with experience not only in DMD but also in techniques of communication. If at all possible, a specialist nurse (the Muscular Dystrophy Campaign family care officers) should also be present at the consultation or visit the family at home shortly after the diagnosis. This is helpful not only to introduce the family to various nonmedical issues (ranging from support at school to disability allowance), but also because it usually takes a long time, often many years, for families to fully understand the implications of a diagnosis like DMD. These professionals can therefore provide important additional information to families, with a feedback to the physicians, by performing home visits after the diagnosis has been made, and advising the family on practical matters such as home modifications.

In order for families to be fully informed of the different problems encountered at different stages of the disease, but also of the various solutions and help that is available, we found it very helpful to run clinics entirely dedicated to DMD patients and focused on specific problems that characterize a particular stage of the disorder. In the ambulant phase children are followed in a dedicated clinic, in which they are recruited for the rehabilitation programme using callipers. Following their loss of independent ambulation, patients are channelled to a combined neuromuscular/orthopaedic clinic where the issue of scoliosis is discussed and individuals are given the opportunity to interact with other patients who have already undergone surgical correction of the spine. In the later stages of the disease, patients with respiratory problems are channelled to a dedicated combined neuromuscular/respiratory clinic for ventilated individuals. Bereavement counselling is offered to all families following the demise of the affected individual. With this pragmatic and dedicated approach, in which the key physician and his or her own team also act as counsellors to the family, informing them of both the problems and solutions available, serious psychological problems are rare. Depression may, however, still develop, especially in adolescents. These cases should be referred to an experienced clinical psychologist or, if required, to a psychiatrist aware of the problems of DMD.

Educational and social needs

The first question to be answered is whether an affected boy may require special schooling. In a few cases associated with severe mental handicap this may be indicated when the parents find management difficult. In most cases, however, boys can derive considerable benefit from attending a normal school where the teachers can be very helpful once the problem has been explained. The several problems that may affect a boy's educational ability include progressive motor difficulties that make acquisition of new skills more difficult and frequent absence from school with declining physical condition. Affected boys also tire easily and may lack initiative and motivation.

Attention should focus on a boy's positive abilities. A proportion will be academically orientated. But their physical incapacity by the time they reach senior school can present a serious problem, and further education and employment prospects are limited but are now being increasingly recognized and addressed. Several of our patients, since the availability of night-time ventilatory support, have completed university degrees. Others work part-time as information technology officers and engineers. Some patients are artistically inclined. Over the years one of us has made a collection of drawings and paintings by patients, and their skill and ability is frequently a source of admiration.

As the disease progresses and boys become confined to a wheelchair, day schools that cater specially for the physically handicapped can be an attractive proposition. In such an environment they will feel less isolated and more able to share feelings and emotions with fellow sufferers. Most parents prefer to have their child in a day school with other handicapped children rather than in an institution away from home.

At home consideration should be given to the time when the DMD patient will be unable to walk unaided and appropriate plans made. Ramps to take a wheelchair may be required. A ground floor bedroom/study is ideal, with TV, hi-fi, computer, and other devices of his choosing. In this way he will have a place that he can consider his private sanctum in which to entertain friends and be on his own if he chooses.

There are a vast array of aids, including wheelchairs, available for the physically handicapped. In several countries including Britain some of these can be obtained through the National Health Service at no cost to the family. It would not be appropriate to deal with these matters here. However, there are several publications that are of considerable practical value and provide information not only on aids but also addresses of where to seek help and advice: these can be obtained through the national support groups, whose addresses are provided in Appendix H.

Drug therapy

The assessment of the possible therapeutic benefits of a drug in DMD presents a number of problems that have to be considered. Very few drug trials in the past have been properly designed.

Early drug trials

Over the last 70 years there have been many drug trials in DMD. Some of the drugs that have been tried and the basis for their use are summarized in Table 13.4. Many of the early studies were ill designed. Often an initial study claiming benefits for a particular drug was subsequently refuted by a better designed and better controlled study.

Table 13.4 Drugs (arranged alphabetically) used in various therapeutic trials in DMD

Drug	Basis for use	Trial
Allopurinol	Increases nucleotide formation believed to be depleted in dystrophic muscle	1976
Amino acids	Deficiency of muscle proteins	1953
Aminoglycoside	Read-through of stop codons	2001
Anabolic steroids	Anabolic effect	1955
Aspirin, propranolol, etc.	Counteract proposed defect in biogenic amine metabolism	1977
Azathioprine	Immunosuppression	1993
Calcium blockers	Reduce muscle intracellular calcium	1982
Catecholamines	Counteract proposed defect in muscle sympathetic innervation	1930
Coenzyme Q	Possible benefit in murine dystrophy	1974
Creatine	Deficiency of muscle creatine	2000
Cyclosporin	Immunosuppression	1993
Dantrolene	Inhibit release of calcium from sarcoplasmic reticulum	1983
Digitalis and other cardiac glycosides	Prevent progressive cardiomyopathy	1963
Glycine	Stimulate muscle creatine synthesis	1932
Growth hormone	Anabolic effect	1973
Growth hormone inhibitor	Growth hormone deficiency ameliorates disease	1984
Ketoacids	Reduce muscle protein degradation	1982
Leucine	Increases protein synthesis	1984
Nucleotides (e.g. Laevadosin)	Replacement of nucleotides believed to be depleted in dystrophic muscle	1960

Table 13.4 *Continued*

Drug	Basis for use	Trial
Oestrogens	Anabolic effect	1972
Oxandrolone	Anabolic effect	1997
Pancreatic extract	Possible benefit in murine dystrophy	1976
Penicillamine	Possible benefit in avian dystrophy	1977
Prednisolone	Anabolic and immunosupressive effect	1974
Protease inhibitors	Possible benefit in murine dystrophy	1984
Superoxide dismutase	Removal of superoxide radicals associated with membrane damage	1980
Testosterone	Anabolic effect	1955
Thyroxine	Thyroxine depresses SCK	1964
Vasodilators	Counteract proposed defect in muscle microcirculation	1963
Vitamin B$_6$	Vitamin B$_6$-deficient rats develop myopathy	1940
Vitamin E	Vitamin E-deficient animals develop myopathy	1940
Zinc	Membrane 'stabilizer'	1986

Evaluation of drug trials

A detailed critical review of the many past therapeutic trials in DMD was carried out in 1980, and a system devised of awarding a 'quality score' for each report, with a point for each of the following criteria: careful selection and definition of cases; adequate controls; objective ('blind') study; assessment other than by simple clinical ratings; and for a trial lasting longer than 2 years. Of 34 trials published, not one was awarded five points, and in half there was no score at all, which means that even the definition of the cases studied was not clear (Table 13.5). Trials with a score of less than three are seriously flawed, and have the danger of raising false hopes in both the patient and his family.

Design of drug trials

There are a number of general points to be considered in designing a DMD drug trial. Patients must be carefully selected on the basis of accepted clinical, biochemical, and genetic diagnostic criteria for the disease. The inclusion of patients with BMD, for example, might give the mistaken impression of slowing the course of the disease. The patients should also be old enough and intelligent enough to cooperate and yet still be ambulant. Ideally, they should therefore be aged between 5 and 10 years. The trial should be 'blind', unless the nature of the treatment (for example, surgery) or the occurrence of unusual

Table 13.5 Scoring of 34 drug trials in DMD (1940–79)*

Score	Number of trials
0	17
1	7
2	3
3	3
4	4
5	0

* Data from Dubowitz and Heckmatt (1980).

side-effects makes this impossible. Ideally, it should be double-blind with neither the patient and his family, nor the investigator, knowing who is taking the drug and who is taking a placebo. It may be difficult to convince parents of the value of this method because if they already believe the drug could be effective it would mean in some cases denying the possible benefits of treatment for the duration of the trial. For this reason a cross-over double-blind study has an advantage, and also requires fewer patients. Others have used 'natural history controls' for comparisons, that is, data collected from known cases over a period of time. The placebo must have the same appearance, texture, and taste as the drug. Furthermore, the effects of the drug may take some time to wear off (the so-called 'wash-out' effect) and so vitiate the results of a cross-over study.

If there are likely to be clear side-effects this would invalidate a double-blind study, and if they could be serious then it is essential that a very carefully monitored pilot study should be carried out initially (so called phase 1 trial). In any trial of new drugs or some form of gene therapy, a phase 1 trial nowadays is mandatory.

The possible beneficial effects may be assessed in regard to prolonged survival, prolonged ambulation, or the slowed or arrested progression of muscle weakness. Since changes in muscle strength will be evident first, most emphasis has been placed on this aspect of the problem (Table 13.6). Details of the scoring and grading systems are given in Appendices B–F. Because there is a subjective element in determining muscle strength, and to some extent functional ability, these are best assessed by one examiner. There is also value in using an ergometer (myometer, dynamometer). One that we currently use is the handheld, sensitive, dead-beat electronic device produced by CITEC, B.V., The Netherlands. The unit has a pressure pad and a digital read-out display that indicates the maximum force applied by the examiner in resisting the actual contraction of the patient's muscles. The operating range is 0.1–30 kg and it has a repeatability error of less than 1 per cent (Fig. 13.8).

Table 13.6 Methods for assessing the possible beneficial effects of a drug in DMD

Muscle strength
MRC grading (0–5)
Ergometry (kg)
Respiratory muscle strength
Functional ability
Vignos grade (1–10)
Hammersmith motor ability score (0–40)
'CIDD' grade for upper limbs (1–6)
Biochemical
SCK
Urinary creatine/creatinine, 3-methylhistidine, dimethylarginines
Muscle pathology and dystrophin expression

In recent years several investigators have measured various biochemical parameters as a means of assessing any possible improvement. Urinary excretion studies are obviously more acceptable than repeated blood sampling though the former require to be very carefully controlled for age, sex, and diet. There is little value in repeated muscle biopsies to evaluate morphological changes, because of the marked variability of pathology due to muscle sampling. A muscle biopsy for dystrophin analysis might, however, be required in drug trials focused on replacement or upregulation of muscle proteins (such as dystrophin or utrophin, for example).

Statistical considerations

A drug trial should be designed in such a way as to avoid errors of suggesting a beneficial effect when none exists or, alternatively, concluding that there is no effect when in fact the drug arrests or slows the disease process. To detect a therapeutic effect that is small, such as a gradual slowing of the disease process, requires a prolonged trial involving a large number of patients. Conversely, a marked therapeutic effect would be detectable in a shorter time and would need fewer individuals. In this regard a helpful parameter to be determined is the so-called power of the trial. If the rate of decline in untreated boys is r_1 (with a standard deviation, SD) and in treated boys is r_2, then the *standard difference* (delta, Δ) is

$$\Delta = (r_1 - r_2)/\text{SD}.$$

The power of a trial is the probability of detecting a difference in the two rates that is statistically significant ($p < 0.05$) and can be calculated for different numbers of individuals and for trials of different durations. Based on data

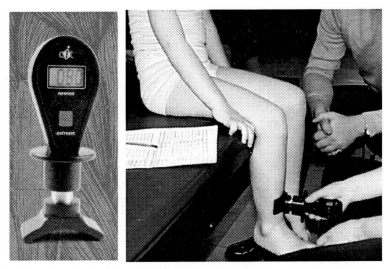

Fig. 13.8 Example of a handheld myometer and its use to evaluate knee extension in a child with DMD.

from 114 untreated boys with DMD followed for a year, power curves have been derived by Brooke *et al.* (1983). These investigators found that the rate of decline in untreated boys was 0.4 units (of muscle strength) per year (SD, 0.39). If after a year a drug slowed the disease to 25 per cent of its original rate of progression, then

$$\Delta = (0.4 - 0.1)/0.39 = 0.77$$

To detect such a difference with a 95 per cent probability would require a study involving at least 40 individuals in each group. On the other hand, if a drug actually arrested the progression of the disease, about 25 individuals in each group would be required (Fig.13.9).

By using more than one set of measurements, the power of a trial study can be increased, thereby decreasing the number of individuals needed and/or the duration of the trial. However, the rate of progression is clearly not the same in all boys. It might therefore be best to consider each boy as being his own control by comparing rates of progression before and after treatment. Alternatively, groups of boys may be compared who, prior to a trial, showed similar rates of progression.

Taking into account the 'power' of a study, the criteria of a good trial in DMD should be:

♦ inclusion only of patients with a clearly established diagnosis of the disease;

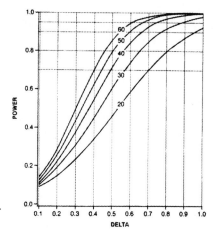

Fig. 13.9 Power curves ($p < 0.05$, one-tail) for drug trials lasting a year for various values of the standard difference (delta). (From Brooke *et al.* (1983) with permission.)

- carefully matched control group;
- 'blind' study;
- assessment by several different methods;
- determination of an acceptable 'power' level and therefore the number of individuals to be studied and the duration of the trial.

The assumption underlying the discussion so far is that quite a large number of patients will be involved in a study. Each individual investigator, however, is unlikely to have access to many patients and therefore collaboration between different centres is necessary, to produce data for a so-called 'multi-centre trial'. Uniformity is then essential, both in the design and execution of the trial, particularly with regard to clinical assessment of the possible effects of a drug. The alternative is to study smaller groups of patients but then, as we have seen, only a comparatively large effect would be detected (Table 13.7).

A useful overview of problems involved in drug trials in DMD can be found in *Muscle and Nerve* (Volume 8, pp. 451–92, 1985), which gives the proceedings of a 1984 colloquium sponsored by the Muscular Dystrophy Association of America. Some other issues have been discussed at an ENMC workshop on therapeutic trials in DMD (Dubowitz *et al.* 2000).

Recent drug trials: glucocorticoids

No curative pharmacological treatment is yet available for DMD but, of all the medications studied so far, glucocorticoids appear to be the most effective in slowing down the disease process. The precise mechanism by which glucocorticoids increase strength in DMD is not known, especially considering their

Table 13.7 Numbers (rounded off) of individuals (controls and treated) required in a randomized trial where there is a 95 per cent probability ('power') of detecting a significant difference ($p < 0.05$; $p < 0.01$) for various values of Δ. In each case numbers are roughly four times the required number for a cross-over trial

Δ	One-tail		Two-tail	
	$p < 0.05$	$p < 0.01$	$p < 0.05$	$p < 0.01$
0.1	2 165	3 154	2 599	3 563
0.2	541	788	650	891
0.4	135	197	162	223
0.6	60	88	72	99
0.8	34	49	41	56
1.0	22	31	26	36
1.2	15	22	18	25
1.4	11	16	13	18
1.6	8	12	10	14
1.8	7	10	8	11
2.0	5	8	6	9

negative effect on normal skeletal muscle (steroid myopathy). Among the possible effects in dystrophic muscle are inhibition of muscle proteolysis, stimulatory effect on myoblast proliferation, anti-inflammatory/immunosuppressive effect with a decrease in muscle T cells, and muscle fibres focally invaded by lymphocytes.

There are now more than two decades of experience with these drugs and the individual studies are listed in Table 13.8. The most commonly used steroid preparations used are prednisone, its hydroxylated form prednisolone (equipotent in glucorticoid effect to prednisone), and deflazacort, an oxazoline derivative of prednisolone. One mg prednisone is equivalent in anti-inflammatory (glucocorticoid) effect to 1.2 mg deflazacort. This latter drug has the advantage of having a lower incidence of weight gain, but other side-effects are similar to those of prednisolone and, in addition, an increased incidence of cataracts has been reported in patients treated with this drug when compared to prednisolone.

Since all these studies have used different steroids or regimens and although the overall results seem to suggest a slowing of the disease process, at least in the short term, there is a need for a large coordinated study using the same

Table 13.8 Glucocorticoid trials in DMD

Authors[†]	Design	N	Age (years)	Glucocorticoid regimen	Treatment period	Outcome	Comments
Drachman 1974	Open	14	4–10.5	Prednisone 2 mg/kg/day for 3 months; then 2/3 dose on alternate days	3 weeks–28 months	Improvement	Side effects in 4
Siegel 1974	Double blind	14	6–9	Prednisone 5 mg/kg alternate days	24 months	No benefit	
Brooke 1987	Open	33	5–15	Prednisone 1.5 mg/kg/day	6 months	Improvement	6 Drop-outs
DeSilva 1987	Open	16	3–10	Prednisone 2 mg/kg/day for 3 months; then 2/3 dose on alternate days	1–11 years	Walking prolonged by 2 years	Excessive weight gain in 12; cataracts in 2
Mendell 1989	Randomized double blind	103	5–15	Prednisone 0.75 mg/kg/day Prednisone 1.5 mg/kg/day	6 months	Improved at 3 months; then stabilization	30% boys had more than 20% weight gain
Fenichel 1991	Double blind	103	5–15	Prednisone 1.25 mg/kg/alternate day Prednisone 2.5 mg/kg/alternate day	6 months	Improved at 3 months	Similar side effects on daily and alternate day regimes
Fenichel 1991b	Open	92	5–15	Prednisone 0.75 mg/kg/day	2 years	Stabilization for 2 years; prednisone 0.65 mg/kg/day least effective dose	Cataracts in 10; glycosuria in 10; significant weight gain
Griggs 1991	Randomized	99	5–15	Prednisone 0.3 mg/kg/day Prednisone 0.75 mg/kg/day	6 months	Strength improved at 10 days	30% boys had more than 20% weight gain
Mesa 1991	Double blind	28	5–11	Deflazacort 1 mg/kg/day	9 months	Improved till 6 months; then stable	35% cushingoid; no significant weight gain
Griggs 1993	Randomized	107	5–15	Prednisone 0.75 mg/kg/day Azathioprine 2.5 mg/kg/day	18 months 12 months	Strength and function improved	No additional benefit of azathioprine
Sansome 1993	Open	32	6–14	Prednisolone 0.75 mg/kg/day, for 10 days/months (10 days on 20 days off)	18 months	Strength improved at 6 months, slow decline at 18months	Less side-effects, but 26% boys had more than 20% weight gain

Table 13.8 *Continued*

Authors[†]	Design	N	Age (years)	Glucocorticoid regimen	Treatment period	Outcome	Comments
Angelini 1994	Randomized	28	6.5–9	Deflazacort 2 mg/kg/alternate days	24 months	Stabilization of strength	70% had >20% weight gain; 1 pathological fracture
Backman 1995	Double blind cross-over	37	4–19	Prednisone 0.3 mg/kg/day	12 months	Stabilization for 1 year	Weight gain in 29%
Bonifati 2000	Randomized	18	5–14	Prednisolone 0.75 mg/kg/day Deflazacort 0.9 mg/kg/day	1 year	Prednisolone and deflazacort equally effective	Weight gain more significant in prednisolone group
Biggar 2001	Open	30	7–15	Deflazacort 0.9 mg/kg/day	3.8 years (± SD 1.5)	Ambulation prolonged; FVC preserved	Cataracts in 30%
Reitter 1995 (data reported in Dubowitz 2000)	Double blind	100	5–till ambulant	Prednisolone 0.75 mg/kg/day Deflazacort 0.9 mg/kg/day	2 years	Muscle function stabilized	Excessive weight gain in prednisolone group; cataracts in 27% of deflazacort group

* Taken with permission from Manzur (2001).

† Full references can be found in Manzur (2001).

steroid and with the same regime to determine if there might also be any possible long-term benefit. One of the authors has used glucocorticoids at the time of the functional deterioration of children with DMD, using a treatment regime that minimizes the long-term side-effects (0.75 mg prednisolone 10 days on and 10 days off).

Growth hormone inhibitors

Growth hormone inhibitors were proposed following a report in the 1980s of a family with DMD in which the eldest affected boy was much less severely affected than his brothers but who also suffered from growth hormone deficiency (Fig. 13.10). One of us has also seen a sporadic case with DMD and growth hormone deficiency with no dystrophin expression in muscle who walked until the age of 18 years. This led to the suggestion that treatment with growth hormone inhibitors might be effective in DMD. Unfortunately, this has not proved to be so. However, these observations do raise a number of intriguing questions regarding the role of growth hormone in the evolution of the disease process.

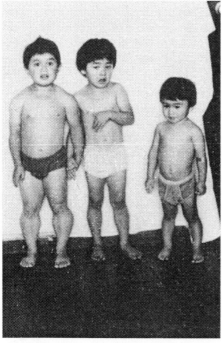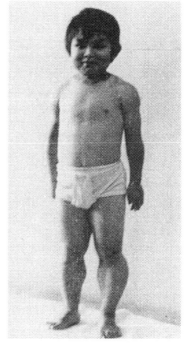

Fig. 13.10 (Left) A boy with DMD and growth hormone deficiency aged 13 and his two younger affected brothers aged 5 and 3. (Right) Proband aged 18. (Reproduced by kind permission of Dr. Mayana Zatz.)

Oxandrolone

A pilot study in 1997 of oxandrolone (an anabolic steroid) in boys with DMD suggested some possible improvement in muscle strength compared with natural history controls. But further double-blind studies have failed to confirm this and oxandrolone cannot be recommended.

Azathioprine and cyclosporin

The mechanism of action of glucocorticoids is unknown but, in view of their immunosuppressive role, other immunosuppressive drugs have been tried, including azathioprine. It was tested in a randomized, controlled trial of prednisolone and azathioprine but failed to have a beneficial effect.

A beneficial effect of cyclosporin on strength (tetanic force and maximum voluntary contraction strength in the tibialis anterior muscle) has been documented after 2 months of cyclosporin therapy but this positive effect was largely lost following a further 2 months wash-out phase. Unfortunately, no functional benefit was assessed and no further studies have been reported.

Creatine

Creatine is converted to phosphocreatine in the muscle where it provides energy in the form of adenosine triphosphate. A modest increase was reported in an early study but it now seems that creatine is unlikely to have any significant effect on the clinical course of DMD.

Aminoglycosides

The administration of gentamycin has been reported to restore dystrophin expression in skeletal muscles of *mdx* mice. The mechanism of action of this aminoglycoside antibiotic is to cause misreading of the RNA code, allowing insertion of alternative amino acids at the site of stop codons. This therefore can theoretically induce a read-through of nonsense mutations. The application of this approach to DMD is limited, as only a minority of patients carry stop codons in the dystrophin gene and trials of the antibiotic in affected boys have been disappointing. Furthermore, this antibiotic has serious oto-nephrotoxic side-effects. Possibly another antibiotic with the same molecular effct but less toxicity might prove beneficial (for example, negamicin).

Gene replacement therapies

Myoblast transfer

The interest in this field was initially derived from the observation that the injection of normal myoblasts into the muscle of dystrophic *mdx* mice rendered many of the fibres in the vicinity of the injection dystrophin-positive. Presumably, the normal myoblasts fused with the host muscle fibres. In the early 1990s some investigators reported having obtained similar results in children with DMD. However, several carefully conducted and extensive studies conducted on a number of boys followed in different centres in the USA and in Canada have concluded that myoblast transplant is not clinically effective in DMD.

This is likely to be partly due to the immune rejection of donor myoblasts (usually from the father) so that after a few months there are no donor-derived dystrophin-positive fibres and virtually no donor-derived nuclei. Other major limitations of this approach would be the difficulties in obtaining cultured myoblasts in sufficient quantities for treatment, and the problem of targeting multiple muscles, including the respiratory and cardiac muscles.

While there does not appear to be any value in myoblast transfer, studies on bone marrow- or muscle-derived stem cells have generated increased interest and enthusiasm (see below).

Gene therapy

Much has been written on the possibility of treating hereditary diseases by gene therapy, and various strategies are being considered using different delivery systems, including viral vectors (for example, DNA adenoviruses or RNA retroviruses) and direct gene transfer. The technical difficulty of each of these approaches is considerable and largely unresolved. In the case of DMD, problems are compounded by the immense size of the dystrophin gene that has to be transferred, limiting the choice of the viral vectors available.

A large number of experiments have been carried out in the *mdx* mice using an adenoviral vector, which has the advantage of being able to contain the entire cDNA of dystrophin. These studies have shown an excellent capability of transfecting individual muscles following direct injection. However, there is significant immune reaction towards the viral vector itself. Moreover, and in common with all gene replacement approaches, there is also some concern for the immunogenicity of dystrophin *per se*, as this molecule will not be recognized as 'self' in DMD patients who have never produced dystrophin. The immune reaction to dystrophin and the viral vector can be overcome by the administration of immunosuppressive drugs. More encouraging results in terms of viral immunogenicity have been achieved by using the adeno-associated virus (AAV), of which different serotypes exist. The AAV is non-pathogenic and is also very efficient in muscle transfection. One limitation is the inability of AAV to package the entire dystrophin cDNA. There are also some technical difficulties related to the production of large quantities of the virus for possible therapy in DMD. Regarding the first point, several authors have exploited the observation that some BMD patients have a mild phenotype despite large in-frame deletions removing nearly 50 per cent of the coding region. A mild BMD phenotype has been reported, for example, in patients with a deletion of exons 16–48 confirming that a large part of the rod domain appears dispensable, as long as the N-and C-termini of dystrophin are retained. In view of the limited immunogenicity of the AAV, this 'mini-dystrophin gene' appears a promising approach. Obviously, the efficiency of the transfection will have to be improved in order to compensate for the fact that the truncated dystrophin molecule is less mechanically efficient compared to the 'normal' dystrophin molecule.

Furthermore, a viral transfer system may not be necessary. Studies have been performed using direct plasmid DNA injection in muscle. These studies followed from earlier observations that injection of plasmid DNA or RNA directly into mouse skeletal muscle can result in significant expression of reporter genes in muscle cells and no special delivery system is necessary. With regard to the transfer of the dystrophin gene, a human dystrophin plasmid cDNA is expressed in transfected cell cultures as well as in *mdx* mouse muscle after being injected intramuscularly. While the efficiency of the original studies was very low, with only about 1 per cent of muscle fibres expressing dystrophin, more recently the efficiency has been significantly improved. This technique certainly offers a method of possibly correcting the gene defect directly. The advantages of this approach are the very limited immunogenicity of the plasmid itself and the absence of limitations related to the size of the transfected cDNA (so that the full-length dystrophin cDNA can be used). The main disadvantage is the need to inject individual muscles repeatedly (as the plasmid behaves as an episome and does not integrate into the muscle nuclei). Possibly an intra-arterial delivery system will help to overcome some of these difficulties.

This approach of direct gene therapy could offer hope of possibly correcting myocardial dysfunction in DMD, although multiple and repeated injections may be necessary and any central nervous system involvement would be unaffected by this regimen.

The possibility of dystrophin gene correction using antisense oligonucleotides or with chimeric DNA/ RNA oligonucleotides is currently receiving attention. These approaches are usually referred as to 'oligonucelotide-mediated gene therapy'. The most studied of these approaches is the use of antisense oligonucleotides targeted against acceptor or donor splice sites of the dystrophin gene. The idea is to modify the physiological splicing of the dystrophin gene and so create 'functional in-frame deletions' in patients with out-of frame deletions or stop codons located in an exon. These methods were initially developed in the *mdx* mouse, which carries a point mutation in exon 23. Various investigators have attempted to induce skipping of exon 23, which carries the deleterious mutation, and the creation of a functional in-frame deletion by targeting the donor or acceptor splice site of this exon. The results, initially *in vitro* (that is, in muscle cell cultures of the *mdx*) but more recently *in vivo*, have been encouraging. This approach has also been applied to *mdx* cardiomyocyte cultures, although the efficiency appears to be lower when compared to skeletal muscle.

A similar approach has been attempted in DMD patients carrying an exon 45 deletion, using an antisense oligoribonucleotide targeted against splicing enhancer sequences located in exon 46. Deletion of exon 45 is an out-of-frame deletion and usually results in DMD. Exon 46 contains a purine-rich sequence that has been shown to regulate splicing of exon 46. These sequences have been named 'splicing enhancer sequences' and targeted antisense oligonlucletoides against them have been shown to increase the splicing of exon 46. This eventually results in a 'functional larger deletion' of exons 45 and 46 with restoration of the reading frame of dystrophin mRNA and dystrophin production (see Fig. 13.11). This approach was recently found to be successful in muscle cell cultures from a DMD patient. Other dystrophin exons carry apparent splicing enhancer sequences (for example, exons 43, 44, 46, 50, and 51). Therefore this approach has the potential to be of value in children with other relatively common deletions.

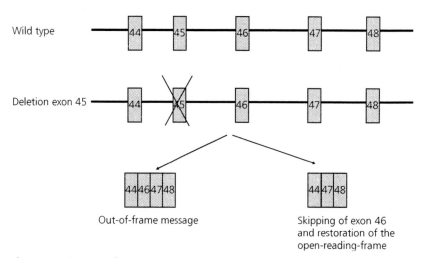

Fig. 13.11 Skipping of exon 46 and restoration of the open reading frame.

One of the major difficulties of this and similar approaches (such as the chimeric DNA/RNA olignoucleotide approach) is the likely need for a systemic delivery.

Stem cell therapy

Stem cells with the potential of developing into muscle cells can be obtained from bone marrow, umbilical blood, or even the early embryo. There is a possibility that such stem cells might prove to be another approach to the treatment of DMD. For example, bone marrow (haemopoietic) stem cells from normal mice have been shown to relocate in the muscle of *mdx* mice and to produce dystrophin. Unfortunately, in these experiments the proportion of muscle cells producing dystrophin was very small. Nevertheless, these observations do raise the possibility of the therapeutic potential for DMD of using some form of stem cells.

Upregulation of other genes/proteins

The observation that utrophin, a homologue of dystrophin, can partially compensate for the absence of dystrophin once upregulated in the *mdx* mice has generated a lot of interest in this as a potential treatment strategy for DMD. The idea is to identify drugs that could significantly upregulate the production of utrophin in skeletal muscle. This protein is expressed at the sarcolemma during fetal life but only at the neuromuscular junction in adult muscle. It is believed that the upregulation of its production at the sarcolemma in DMD might compensate for the lack of dystrophin. Another advantage of utrophin is the likely absence of any immune reaction to this protein as it should be recognized as 'self'. Indeed the re-introduction of dystrophin following gene therapy in the *mdx* mice is followed by a strong immune reaction against dystrophin. This does not occur with utrophin since it is physiologically produced in all individuals with DMD.

Studies have also shown that the upregulation of integrin $\alpha7$ (see Fig. 10.1, p. 160) is capable of preventing development of the pathology in the *mdx* mice. Thus, the possibility that some pharmacological agent will be found that will upregulate utrophin, integrin $\alpha7$, or even some other protein and ultimately prove therapeutic in DMD is an attractive one.

Summary and conclusions

Although DMD is not curable, effective treatments are available that can improve the quality of life and survival of affected boys. Paramount is the maintenance of good general health with emphasis on good nutrition and weight control, the prevention of deformities, and the preservation of respiratory function. The development of deformities can be delayed by passive exercises and ambulation can be prolonged with callipers and various other orthoses. Scoliosis is a particularly serious problem because the progressive thoracic deformity restricts adequate pulmonary ventilation and aggravates respiratory problems resulting from weakness of the intercostal muscles. The development of scoliosis can be limited by fitting an appropriate moulded thoracolumbar orthosis, but more effectively by prolonging ambulation and surgical fixation of the spine. However, spinal surgery is a major operation that carries its own complications. Only patients with a definite progressive scoliosis should be considered for this operation. While occasionally patients may develope rhabdomyolysis following a general anaesthetic, this appears to be a rare complication, almost restricted to young children, and can be prevented by avoiding certain muscle relaxants. While for the majority of patients there are no serious anaesthetic or postoperative problems, the anaesthetist and surgeon need to be prepared against these eventualities and careful monitoring of respiratory and cardiac function should be performed before and after any major surgery.

Impaired pulmonary function is the major factor in morbidity and mortality. Over 90 per cent of deaths are due to pulmonary infection and respiratory failure. The preservation of respiratory function can be achieved to an extent by impeding the development of scoliosis. All respiratory infections must be treated vigorously. In the later stages of the disease, assisted ventilation can be helpful in relieving symptoms associated with hypoventilation and may well prolong life.

The psychological effects of the disease on the patient himself as well as on his parents and unaffected sibs cannot be ignored. Open and frequent discussions between all those concerned, including health-care professionals, should be encouraged. The educational needs of affected boys can also raise problems for those who are severely handicapped and may require special care. There are increasing possibilities for those who are highly intelligent to get higher education despite their severe physical handicap.

In recent years there has been considerable interest in the design of drug trials in this disease. Glucocorticoids seem to have a beneficial effect in retarding the progression of the disease at least in the short term. However their use is associated with side-effects, so that these need to be carefully discussed with the family and the affected child. Regimens to limit the incidence of side-effects but still retain a positive effect on disease progression have been devised and are being evaluated in large studies. These studies will also have to demonstrate the long-term benefits of steroids.

Despite early enthusiasm for myoblast transfer, subsequent studies indicate that this approach is not clinically effective. However, gene therapy approaches are now being pursued. Some form of stem cell therapy also offers the possibility of treating the disease.

There are now good reasons to entertain cautious optimism that an effective treatment for DMD may well be found in the not too distant future.

References and further reading

Brooke, M.H., Fenichel, G.M., Griggs, R.C., Mendell, J.R., Moxley, R., Miller, J.P., and Province, M.A. (1983). Clinical investigation in Duchenne dystrophy: 2. Determination of 'power' of therapeutic trials based on the natural history. *Muscle and Nerve* **6**, 91–103.

Dubowitz, V. (1997). 47th ENMC International workshop: treatment of muscular dystrophy, 13–15 Dec 1996, Naarden, The Netherlands. *Neuromuscular Disorders* **7**, 261–7.

Dubowitz V. (2000). 75th ENMC International workshop: Treatment of muscular dystrophy, Baarn 10–12 Dec, 1999. *Neuromuscular Disorders* **10**, 313–20.

Dubowitz, V. and Heckmatt, J. (1980). Management of muscular dystrophy. *British Medical Bulletin* **36**, 139–44.

Dubowitz, V., Hyde, S.A., Scott, O.M., and Goddard, C. (1984). Controlled trial of exercise in Duchenne muscular dystrophy. In *Neuromuscular diseases* (ed. G. Serratice *et al.*), pp. 571–5. Raven Press, New York.

Eagle, M., Baudouin, S.V., Chandler, C., Giddings, D.R., Bullock, R., and Bushby, K. (2002). Survival in Duchenne muscular dystrophy: improvements in life expectancy since 1967 and the impact of home nocturnal ventilation. *Neuromuscul Disord* **12**, 926–9.

Emery, A.E.H. (2000). *Muscular dystrophies: the facts*, 2nd edn. Oxford University Press, Oxford.

Emery, A.E.H. and Pullen, I.M. (eds.) (1984). *Psychological aspects of genetic counselling*. Academic Press, London.

Griffiths, R.D. and Edwards, R.H. (1988). A new chart for weight control in Duchenne muscular dystrophy. *Archives of Disease in Childhood* **63**, 1256–8.

Hyde, S.A. (1984). *The parent's guide to the physicial management of Duchenne muscular dystrophy*. Muscular Dystrophy Group of Great Britain and Northern Ireland, London.

Hyde, S.A., Flytrup, I., Glent, S., Kroksmark, A.K., Salling, B., Steffensen, B.F., Werlauff, U., and Erlandsen, M. (2000). A randomized comparative study of two methods for controlling tendo achilles contracture in Duchenne muscular dystrophy. *Neuromuscular Disorders* **10**, 257–63

Manzur, A.Y. (2001). Medical management and treatment of Duchenne muscular dystrophy. In *The muscular dystrophies* (ed. A.E.H. Emery). Oxford University Press, Oxford.

Rideau, Y., Duport, G., and Delaubier, A. (1986). Premières rémissions reproductibles dans l'évolution de la dystrophie musculaire de Duchenne. *Bull Acad Nat Méd* **170**, 605–610.

Rodillo, E.B., Fernandez-Bermejo, Heckmatt, J.Z., *et al.* (1988). Prevention of rapidly progressive scoliosis in Duchenne muscular dystrophy by prolongation of walking with orthosis. *Journal of Child Neurology* **3**, 269–74.

Siegel, I.M., Miller, J.E., and Ray, R.D. (1968). Subcutaneous lower limb tenotomy in the treatment of pseudohypertrophic muscular dystrophy. *Journal of Bone and Joint Surgery* **50A**, 1437–43.

Simonds, A.K., Muntoni, F., Heather, S., and Fielding, S. (1998). Impact of nasal ventilation on survival in hypercapnic Duchenne muscular dystrophy. *Thorax* **53**, 949–52.

Smith, P.E.M., Calverley, P.M.A., Edwards, R.H.T., Evans, G.A., and Campbell, E.J.M. (1987). Practical problems in the respiratory care of patients with muscular dystrophy. *New England Journal of Medicine* **316**, 1197–205.

Spencer, G.E. and Vignos, P.J. (1962). Bracing for ambulation in childhood progressive muscular dystrophy. *Journal of Bone and Joint Surgery* **44A**, 234–42.

Thompson, C.E. (1999). *Raising a child with a neuromuscular disorder*. Oxford University Press, Oxford.

Vignos, P.J., Spencer, G.E., and Archibald, K.C. (1963). Management of progressive muscular dystrophy of childhood. *Journal of the American Medical Association* **184**, 89–96.

Zellweger, H. (1975). Family counselling in Duchenne muscular dystrophy. In *Recent advances in myology* (ed. W.G. Bradley, D. Gardner-Medwin, and J.N. Walton), pp. 469–71. Excerpta Medica, Amsterdam.

Because of the growing awareness of the importance of physiotherapy in muscular dystrophy, an International Congress on the subject was held in Italy in 1984, the Proceedings of which have now been published in detail (*Cardiomyology*, Volume 3, nos 2–3, 1984). The reader will find therein helpful information including some useful guidelines proposed by the European Alliance of Muscular Dystrophy Associations.

Duchenne's obituary (*Lancet* 1875)

Duchenne (De Boulogne)

(From our Paris Correspondent)

DUCHENNE (DE BOULOGNE), whose death you noticed in your last issue, was born in 1806, and consequently died at the age of about seventy. After having graduated he began practice in Boulogne-sur-Mer, his native place, but soon found this field too narrow for his restless and inventive mind, and for the experiments which he was already conducting, and so he left for Paris, where, during thirty-three years, he led a life of incessant scientific labour.

In 1847 he presented his first memoir to the Academy of Sciences, and up to within a month previous to his death he continued to publish, either in the Transactions of the two Academies or in the *Archives de Médecine*, the results of his experiments and observations. Amongst the most important of his researches are those on the muscular system: the isolated action and synergy of muscles. His studies on the muscles of the face, and on their office in the mechanism and expression of the human visage, are remarkable, and are familiar in France to artists as well as to medical men. But it was especially in his researches on the nervous centres, on the various forms of paralysis, on congenital or developed deformities, that his great qualities of observation manifested themselves. His name will ever be coupled with the history of progressive muscular atrophy, locomotor ataxy (to which Trousseau proposed that the name of 'Duchenne's disease' should be given), glosso-labio-laryngeal paralysis, and, generally, the microscopical anatomy and pathology of the nervous system. His right of priority to the description of certain forms of nervous diseases has been disputed, and with justice; as, for instance, in the case of locomotor ataxy, where Romberg certainly had the precedence. But at the same time, it may be stated that all Duchenne's descriptions and discoveries were original, and the result of his own labours. The writings of Romberg and other foreign savants were at the time unknown in France, not only to Duchenne, but even to the best men having a knowledge of foreign languages.

A great many of his researches were carried on by means of electricity, and in turn they threw light on the uses of this powerful agent, and to Duchenne will redound the honour of having methodically applied electricity to physiological and pathological investigations, and of having scientifically used it for the treatment of disease.

His features were familiar to all who visited habitually the wards of the Paris hospitals. Every morning Duchenne was to be seen in one or other of the hospitals, studying cases, examining specimens, drawing his photographs of microscopical appearances, in which he was extraordinarily skilful. For a long time Duchenne's invariable presence in the wards, his incessant moving about, his ardent interrogation of patients, caused him to be looked upon with a somewhat suspicious and anxious eye by many of the hospital physicians. But his consummate experience of disease, his wonderful keenness and ability in making out a diagnosis in cases of paralysis, the sincerity and earnestness of his manner, the honesty of his proceedings, the authority which he gained by the publication of his original researches, the services which he rendered daily in the wards of the hospitals, brought him the esteem and appreciation of all, and made him a welcome guest everywhere.

He was no orator, and could never have given a lecture on any subject, but he was wonderful at the patient's bedside. Dexterous and nimble in handling his patient, sharp and sensible in his questioning, most striking in the way he got up his data, made out the disease, and gave practical demonstrations of the surety of his diagnosis. Amongst the various instances of this last quality which were related in the hospitals about Duchenne was the fact of his taking patients accounted to be paraplegic out of their beds, and of causing a man to get on their shoulders without their giving way in the slightest.

His patience was extraordinary. He would pursue the investigation of a case for years, never losing sight of it, and following the patient in his peregrinations from hospital to hospital and from house to house, often affording help and means of subsistence. It may be said of Duchenne that under many adverse circumstances—the suspicions of confréres, the disputes as to priority, the difficulty of finding a field of study and experiment, as he had no hospital appointment—his reputation has come out clear and bright, as an honest, hardworking, acute, and ingenious observer, an original discoverer, a skilful professional man, and a kind-hearted, benevolent gentleman.

His various writings have been gathered, and are included in the following important works:— 'Traité de l'Electrisation Localisée' (third edition); 'Le Mécanisme de la Physionomie Humaine'; 'La Physiologie des Mouvements Démontrée à l'aide de l'Expérimentation Electrique'; 'Anatomie du Système Nerveux', 'Orthopédie Physiologique'.

MRC grading of muscle strength (MRC 1943)

	Grade
No contraction	0
Flicker or trace of contraction only	1
Active movement with gravity eliminated	2
Active movement against gravity	3
Active movement against gravity and resistance	4
Normal power	5

Reference

MRC (1943). *Aids to the investigation of peripheral nerve injuries.* MRC War Memorandum no. 7 (2nd edn). HMSO, London.

Appendix C

Swinyard grade (Swinyard *et al.* 1957)

	Grade
Walks with waddling gait and marked lordosis. Elevation activities adequate (climbs stairs and curbs without assistance).	1
Walks with waddling gait and marked lordosis. Elevation activities deficient (needs support for curbs and stairs).	2
Walks with waddling gait and marked lordosis. Cannot negotiate curbs or stairs but can achieve erect posture from standard height chair.	3
Walks with waddling gait and marked lordosis. Unable to rise from a standard height chair	4
Wheelchair independence. Good posture in the chair; can perform all activities of daily living from chair.	5
Wheelchair with dependence. Can roll chair but needs assistance in bed and wheelchair activities.	6
Wheelchair with dependence and back support. Can roll the chair only a short distance; needs back support for good chair position.	7
Bed patient. Can do no activities of daily living without maximum assistance.	8

Reference

Swinyard, C.A., Deaver, G.G., and Greenspan, L. (1957). Gradients of functional ability of importance in rehabilitation of patients with progressive muscular and neuromuscular diseases. *Archives of Physical and Medical Rehabilitation* **38**, 574–9.

Vignos grade (Archibald and Vignos 1959)

	Grade
Walks and climbs stairs without assistance.	1
Walks and climbs stairs with aid of railing.	2
Walks and climbs stairs slowly with aid of railing (over 25 seconds for 8 standard steps).	3
Walks but cannot climb stairs.	4
Walks unassisted but cannot climb stairs or get out of chair.	5
Walks only with assistance or with braces.	6
In wheelchair. Sits erect. Can roll chair and perform bed and wheelchair activities of daily living.	7
In wheelchair. Sits erect. Unable to perform bed and chair activities without assistance.	8
In wheelchair. Sits erect only with support. Able to do only minimal activities of daily living.	9
In bed. Can do no activities of daily living without assistance.	10

Reference

Archibald, K.C. and Vignos, P.J. (1959). A study of contractures in muscular dystrophy. *Archives of Physical and Medical Rehabilitation* **40**, 150–7.

Hammersmith motor ability score (Scott *et al.* 1982)

All movements are attempted and scored:

- 2 for every completed movement;
- 1 for help and/or reinforcement;
- 0 if unable to achieve the movement.

Total possible score = 4.

1. Lifts head.
2. Supine to prone over right.
3. Supine to prone over left.
4. Prone to supine over right.
5. Prone to supine over left.
6. Gets to sitting.
7. Sitting.
8. Gets to standing.
9. Standing.
10. Standing on heels.
11. Standing on toes.
12. Stands on right leg.
13. Stands on left leg.
14. Hops on right leg.
15. Hops on left leg.
16. Gets off chair.
17. Climbing step right leg.
18. Descending step right leg.
19. Climbing step left leg.
20. Descending step left leg.

Reference

Scott, O.M., Hyde, S.A., Goddard, C., and Dubowitz, V. (1982). Quantitation of muscle function in children: a prospective study in Duchenne muscular dystrophy. *Muscle and Nerve* 5, 291–301.

Clinical investigation of Duchenne dystrophy (CIDD) group. Grade for upper limb function (Brooke *et al.* 1983)

	Grade
Starting with arms at the sides, patient can abduct the arms in a full circle until they touch above the head.	1
Can raise arms above head only by flexing the elbow (i.e. shortening the circumference of the movement) or by using accessory muscles.	2
Cannot raise hands above head but can raise an 8 oz glass of water to mouth (using both hands if necessary).	3
Can raise hands to mouth but cannot raise an 8 oz glass of water to mouth.	4
Cannot raise hand to mouth but can use hands to hold pen or pick up pennies from table.	5
Cannot raise hands to mouth and has no useful function of hands.	6

Reference

Brooke, M.H., Fenichel, G.M., Griggs, R.C., *et al.* (1983). Clinical investigation in Duchenne dystrophy: 2. Determination of the 'power' of therapeutic trials based on the natural history. *Muscle and Nerve* **6**, 91–103.

Appendix G

Polymorphisms in the dystrophin gene

Further information can be obtained from the Leiden Muscular Dystrophy pages at www.DMD.NL

Probe name	DXS no.	GenBank	Localization	PIC/HF*
5'DYS-I			3.5 kb 5' Dp427b exon 1	0.61
5'DYS-II	DXS1242	L01538	1.2 kb 5' Dp427b exon 1	0.77
5'DYS-III			3.5 kb 3' Dp427b exon 1	0.59
5'DYS-IV			4.2 kb 3' Dp427b exon 1	0
MP1Q			?	0.08
MP1S			?	?
5'DYS MSA identical with	DXS1243		Dp427m intron 1	0.57
5'-5n1		X75920	Dp427m intron 1	
5'-5n3		X75801	intron 1	0.76
5'DYS MSB			intron 1–11	0.25
5'DYS MSC			intron 1–11	0
5'-5n4		X77678	intron 4–5	0.64
DMDSTR07A	(DXS206)	U60822	22 kb 3' exon 7	0.68
DMDSTR07B	(DXS206)	U60822	23 kb 3' exon 7	0.44
5'-7n4		X77677	intron 25–28	0.52
STR44	DXS1238	M81257	13.8 kb 3' exon 44	0.86
IVS44SK12			50 kb 3' exon 44, . . . bp 5' IVS44SK21	0.38
IVS44SK21		X77644	50 kb 3' exon 44, . . . bp 5' Dp140 promoter/exon 1	0.87
AFM297yd1	DXS1219	Z24187	intron 44	0.59
P20-CA	DXS269	M86524	40 kb 5' exon 45	>0.80
STR45	DXS1237		1.2 kb 3' exon 45	0.89
STR-45.2			. . . kb 3' exon 45	

Continued

Probe name	DXS no.	GenBank	Localization	PIC/HF*
STR48 identical with AFM217xa5	DXS997	Z16983	9 kb 5′ exon 49	0.7
STR49	DXS1236		intron 49	0.93
STR50	DXS1235		intron 50	0.72
AFM234vg7	DXS1067	Z23710	5.5 kb 5′ exon 51	0.6
AFM072zh3	DXS1036	Z23325	intron 51	0.73
DMD1-2c	DXS1241	X55151	intron 55–57	0.51
STR62/63			intron 61–62	
AFM283wg9	DXS1214	Z24023	intron 62–63	0.78
3′–19n8		X75580	3′ of exon 63	0.58
3′DYS MS			in exon 79	0.34
MP1P			in exon 79	0.22
AFM184xg5	DXS992	Z16803	>20 kb 3′ exon 79	0.87
AFM112xf2	DXS985	Z16589	>20 kb 3′ exon 79	0.61

* PIC/HF, PIC value/heterozygosity frequency.

Muscular dystrophy associations and groups in various countries (Emery 2000)

Argentina
CIDIM
Zapiola 740 CP 1426
Buenos Aires

Australia
Muscular Dystrophy Association of
SA Inc.
GPO Box 414
Adelaide SA 5001

Muscular Dystrophy Association of
NSW
GPO Box 9932
Sydney 2001

Muscular Dystrophy Association of
Queensland
PO Box 518
Sunnybank QLD 4109

Muscular Dystrophy Association of
Victoria
PO Box 182
Ascot Vale VIC 3032

Muscular Dystrophy Association of
Tasmania
Flat 4, 16 Hill Street
Bellerive TAS 7018

Muscular Dystrophy Association of
ACT
PO Box 117
Campbell ACT 2601

Muscular Dystrophy Research
Association of Western
Australia
PO Box 328
West Perth WA 6005

Austria
Österreichische Gesellschaft zur
Bekämpfung der
Muskelkrankheiten
Wahringer Görtel 18–20
Postfach 23
A-1097 Wien

Belgium
Vlaamse Vereniging Neuro-
musculaire
Aandoeningen (NeMA)
Hutsepotstraat 50
B–9052 Zwijnaarde

Association Belge contre les
Maladies
Neuromusculaires (ABMM)
Rue de Blanc Bois 2
1360 Perwez

Brazil
Associacão Brasileira de Distrofia
Muscular
Rua do Matão 277
Edificio da Biologia
Cidade Universitária
CEP 05499 São Paulo

Bulgaria
Bulgarian Neuromuscular Diseases
Association (BNDA)
182 Rakovski Street
Sofia

Canada
Muscular Dystrophy Association of
Canada
150 Eglington Avenue E
Suite 400
Toronto M3P 1E8

Muscular Dystrophy Association of
Canada
Ms Elona Brown
460 O'Connor Street
Suite 215
Ottawa
Ontario K1S 511S

Society for Muscular Dystrophy
Information
PO Box 479
Bridgewater
Nova Scotia B4V 2X6

Croatia
Savez Drustava Distroficara
Hrvatske
10000 ZAGREB, Nova Ves 44
Republika Hrvatska

Cyprus
Muscular Dystrophy Association of
Cyprus
PO Box 3462
Nicosia CY 1638

Czech Republic
Asociace Muskularnich Dystrofiku
v CR
Petyrkova 1953/24
148–00 Praha 4

Denmark
Muskelsvindfonden
Kongsvang Alle 23
DK–8000 Arhus C

EAMDA (Secretariat)
European Alliance of Muscular
Dystrophy Associations
7–11 Prescott Place
London SW4 6BS
Tel: (44)020 7720 8055
Fax: (44)020 7498 8963
E-mail: mail@eamda.sonnet.co.uk

The EAMDA Secretariat can
supply updated listings of all
European member associations
along with their telephone, fax,
and E-mails

ENMC
European Neuromuscular Centre
Lt. Gen.van Heutszlaan 6
NL–3743 JN Baarn
The Netherlands

Estonia
Eesti Lihasehaigete Selts
Energia 8
11316 Tallinn

Finland
Lihastautiliitto R. Y.
Lantinen Pitkakatu 35
SF–20100 Turku

France
Association Francaise contre les
Myopathies (AFM)
1, Rue de l'Internationale
B.P. 59
91002 Evry

Germany
Deutsche Gesellschaft fur
Muskelkranke e V (DGM)
Im Moos 4
79112 Freiburg

Hungary
Hungarian Neuromuscular
Disorders Association
c/o Dr Herczegfalvi/Heim Pal
Children's Hospital
Ulloi ut 86
1089 Budapest

India
Indian Muscular Dystrophy
Association (IMDA)
21–136 Batchupet
Machilipatnam
521 001 (A.P.)

Ireland
Muscular Dystrophy Ireland
Carmichael House, North Brunswick
Street
Dublin 7

Israel
Muscle Disease Association of
Israel
PO Box 1491
61014 Tel Aviv

Italy
Unione Italiana Lotta alla Distrofia
Musculare (UILDM)
Via Gozzadani 7
20148 Milano M1

Unione Italiana Lotta alla Distrofia
Musculare (UILDM)
Via P.P. Vergerio 17
I–35126 Padova

Japan
Muscular Dystrophy Association of
Japan
2-2-8 Nishi-waseda
Shinjuku-ku
Tokyo 162

National Centre for Nervous,
Mental, and Muscular Disorders
Kodaira
Tokyo 187

Lithuania
Lithuanian Neuromuscular
Association
Eiveniu-2
3007 Kaunas

Malta
Muscular Dystrophy Group of Malta
4 Gzira Road
Gzira GZR 04

Moldova Republic
Moldavian Myopathy Association
Street Bulgara 24/B2
Chisinau

The Netherlands
Vereniging Spierziekten
Nederland (VSN)
Lt. Gen. van Heutszlaan 6
NL–3743 JN Baarn

New Zealand
Muscular Dystrophy Association of
New Zealand
PO Box 23–047
Papatoetoe
Auckland

Norway
Foreningen for Muskelsyke
Postboks 4568–Torshov
N–0404 Oslo

Pakistan
Ma Ayshe Memorial Centre
SNPA–22, Block 7/8
Nr. Commercial Area
KMCHS
Karachi

Poland
Towarzystwo Zwalczania Chorob
Miesni
ul. Sw. Bonifacego 10
02–914 Warsaw

Portugal
APMG/DNM
Hospital de Santa Maria
Centro Estudos Egas Moniz
Av. Prof. Egas Moniz
P–1699 Lisboa

Romania
Asociatia Distroficilor Muscular din
Romania (ADMR)
Str. Bailor 197
4017–Vilcele
Jud. Covasna

Russia
The Interregional Association of
Assistance to People
Suffering Neuromuscular Diseases
(The Hope)
Rublevskoe Shosse, d.44, k.
1, kv. 162
Moscow 121609

Slovakia
Organizacia Muskularnych
Dystrofikov v SR
Banselova 4
82104 Bratislava

Slovenia
Drustvo Misicno obolelih Slovenije
Linhartova 1-III
61109 Ljubljana

South Africa
Muscular Dystrophy Research
Foundation of South Africa
PO Box 1535
Pinegowrie 2123

Muscular Dystrophy Research
Foundation – Cape Branch
PO Box 126
Constantia 7848

Spain
Association Espanola de
Enfermedades
Musculares (ASEM)
Gran Via Corts Catalanes 562
08011 Barcelona

Sweden
Neurologiskt Handikappades
Riksforbund (NHR)
Box 3284
103 65 Stockholm

Rorelsehindrade Barn och
Ungdomar (RBU)
Box 6607
113 84 Stockholm

Switzerland
Schweizerische Gesellschaft fur
Muskelkranke (SGMK)
Kanzleistrasse 80
CH–8004 Zurich

Association Suisse Romande contre
la Myopathie (ASRM)
Ch.de la Traverse 12
PO Box 179
CH–1170 Aubonne

Turkey
Turkiye Kas Hastaliklari Dernegi
Hatboyu cd.No.12, Yesilkoy
34800 Istanbul

United Kingdom
Muscular Dystrophy Campaign
(MDC)
7–11 Prescott Place
London
SW4 6BS
Website: www.muscular-dystrophy.org

Mobility International
228 Borough High Street
London
SE1 1JX

Motor Neurone Disease Association
61 Derngate
Northampton
NN1 1 UE

Ukraine
Ukrainian Muscular Dystrophy
Association (ERB)
Shevchenko str., 55/11
290039 LVIV

United States of America
Muscular Dystrophy Association of
America
3300 East Sunrise Drive
Tucson
AZ 85718–3208

Uruguay
Asociacion Uruguaya de
Aldeas Infantiles SOS
Montevideo

WAMDA
World Alliance of Muscular
Dystrophy Associations
13 Place de Rungis
75013 Paris

Yugoslavia, Federal Republic
Savez Distroficara Jugoslavije
Maksima Gorkog 28a
11000 Beograd

Reference

Emery, A.E.H. (2000). Muscular *dystrophy: the facts*, 2nd edn. Oxford University Press, Oxford.

Index